"Putting the words pirate and care together already produces a spark of excitement, asking us to imagine how we are going to make the world together. A world in which what are often separate practices, and languages about practices, can come together. Where abolition, hacking, the commons, queerness, and repair are connected. Where, as good feminists, we concern ourselves with the work and play that sustains us, in and against the empires of extraction. A most nourishing and encouraging little book."

—McKenzie Wark, author of
A Hacker Manifesto and *Capital is Dead*

"In times of rampant institutionalized cruelty and neglect, and as we witness the increasing commodification, weaponization and criminalization of care, this inspiring and stimulating collection celebrates care's uncompromising radicality—from anonymous everyday solidarity to bold acts of resistance in the face of ruthless repression. *Pirate Care* is a breath of fiery courage against the suffocation of hope."

—María Puig de la Bellacasa, author of *Matters of Care: Speculative Ethics in More Than Human Worlds*

V̄AG ABO ND̲S

Radical pamphlets to fan the flames of discontent
at the intersection of research,
art and activism.

Series editor: Max Haiven

Also available

007

Pirate Care

Acts Against
the Criminalization
of Solidarity

Valeria Graziano, Marcell Mars
and Tomislav Medak

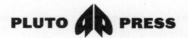

First published 2025 by Pluto Press
New Wing, Somerset House, Strand, London WC2R 1LA
and Pluto Press, Inc.
1930 Village Center Circle, 3-834, Las Vegas, NV 89134

www.plutobooks.com

British Library Cataloguing in Publication Data
A catalogue record for this book is available from the
British Library

ISBN 978 0 7453 4980 0   Paperback
ISBN 978 0 7453 4982 4   PDF
ISBN 978 0 7453 4981 7   EPUB

This book is printed on paper suitable for recycling and
made from fully managed and sustained forest sources.
Logging, pulping and manufacturing processes are
expected to conform to the environmental standards of
the country of origin.

Typeset by Stanford DTP Services, Northampton,
England

Simultaneously printed in the United Kingdom and
United States of America

Contents

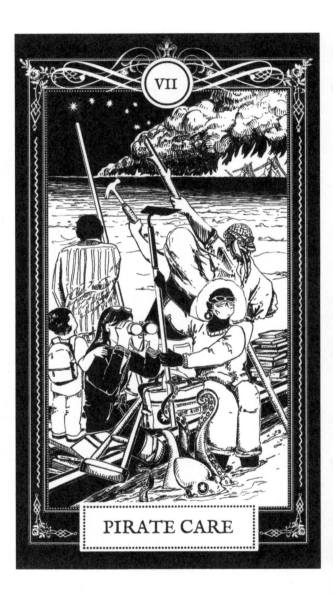

VII

PIRATE CARE

Ouverture
For a Global Mutiny

Three tales from the high seas

Sea-Watch

In June 2019, the coast of Sicily basked in summer's warmth, offering a peaceful contrast to the dire situation aboard *Sea-Watch 3*. Captain Carola Rackete, resolute on the bridge, decided it was time to attempt entry into the port, aware that the men of "Il Capitano" were ready to stop her. Her 53 migrant passengers, rescued from a rubber dinghy 17 days earlier, needed care on land. For two weeks, Italy denied them entry, and psychological stress among the travelers escalated.

At 1:15 am on June 29, Captain Rackete began docking procedures at Lampedusa without authorization. In a video to supporters and the world, she declared, "I know this is risky and that I will probably lose the boat, but the shipwrecked on board are exhausted. I will bring them to safety. Their life is more important than political games." The night air mingled with the scent of diesel, and the low hum of the engine was the only sound as *Sea-Watch 3* approached the port. She informed the port authorities and proceeded. A military patrol boat tried to block the vessel, leading to a collision. Matteo Salvini, Italy's Deputy Prime Minister, later called it "an act of war."

Finally, *Sea-Watch 3* docked, and the relieved migrants disembarked. Some knelt to kiss the ground, others embraced the crew. While thousands die crossing the Mediterranean each year (the official annual death toll of people whom the European Union lets drown regularly surpasses 2,000, but many more go unreported), Rackete was arrested, charged with aiding illegal immigration and resisting a warship, facing up to ten years in prison. Salvini, known as "Il Capitano," condemned her, publicly calling her actions "piracy" and labeling her a "potential murderer," an "outlaw," and a "showoff," as if her actions (perhaps like his) were merely for attention. His fascist rhetoric, steeped in misogyny and xenophobia, painted Rackete as everything a proper white woman shouldn't be: captaining boats, saving lives, defying authority. The far-right's vitriol forced Rackete to go underground for a time. Ultimately, the court ruled in her favor, upholding her duty as a captain to ensure the safety of those on her ship. Rackete's lawyer then sued Salvini for aggravated defamation, accusing him of inciting threats against her.

Women on Waves

On June 11, 2001, two doctors and a nurse sailed out toward Ireland on a Dutch ship equipped as a mobile clinic by the organization Women on Waves. Their mission was to offer reproductive healthcare, including abortion pills, to women in Ireland, where abortion at that time was still illegal.

Women on Waves had discovered a loophole: 12 miles offshore, beyond Ireland's territorial waters, local laws were superseded by the regulations of the flag under which a vessel sails. The clinic on a vessel could legally dispense mifepristone and misoprostol under Dutch law, which allows the termination of a pregnancy up to the 49th day.

The mission stirred international controversy before it even began. Under pressure from Christian parties, the Dutch parliament debated the group's license. Irish authorities sought to block the boat. Women on Waves prepared for potential confrontations, training in security and self-defense.

As they neared Ireland, the excitement and tension of Women on Waves activists mounted.

By the time we arrived in Ireland we had received 80 calls from women requesting abortion services. We did not have nearly enough mifepristone pills on hand to meet this demand . . . All these obstacles forced us to abandon our original plan to provide the abortion pill, which we deeply regretted. Even after it was announced that we would not provide the abortion pill, phone calls kept coming in . . . After five days, 300 women had contacted the ship's hotline. They included women who had been raped, schoolgirls who could not find a feasible excuse to go to England for a couple of days [or] could not pay for childcare . . . and political refugees who did not have the papers to travel . . .[1]

Although they couldn't deliver the abortion pill during this first mission, the women visited the ship and the crew provided other forms of reproductive care, including pregnancy tests, ultrasound scans, and contraceptives.

Women on Waves would go on to organize similar voyages to Poland (2003), Portugal (2004), Spain (2008), Morocco (2012), and Guatemala and Mexico (2017). In Poland, where extreme laws made even discussing abortion a crime (violating the EU Convention on Human Rights), they faced a particularly dramatic reception, with supporters cheering but hostile opponents throwing eggs and paint at the ship and threatening worse. In Portugal, the defense minister sent warships to block the ship, creating an atmosphere of intense repression. Despite the intimidations, Rebecca Gomperts, the founder of Women on Waves, appeared on Portuguese television, casually explaining during her live interview how two widely available pills could be combined to safely terminate pregnancies. Portugal decriminalized abortion two years later.

The work of Women on Waves highlights a grim reality: 73 million women worldwide choose abortion annually, but nearly half of these procedures are unsafe, leading to 150,000 deaths each year, making it one of the leading causes of maternal mortality. Developing countries bear 97 percent of this burden.

Freedom Flotilla

In late August 2008, 44 activists from 17 countries gathered in Cyprus to embark on a daring mission aboard two small ships, *Free Gaza* and *Liberty*, aiming to break Israel's blockade of Gaza. Since 2007 this blockade has isolated over 2 million Palestinians, cutting off essential supplies like food, electricity, and medical supplies. The activists' mission, to provide support directly to Palestinians, was unprecedented—something even governments had not dared to attempt.

The journey was fraught with danger. Israeli navy ships shadowed the ships, jamming their navigation systems. Yet, after more than 30 hours at sea, they reached Gaza on August 23. The sight that met them was overwhelming: thousands of Palestinians gathered, offering a warm, long-repressed welcome.

The activists spent six days in Gaza, visiting hospitals, distributing medicines, and accompanying fishermen to sea to protect them from harassment. When they left on August 29, they brought seven Palestinians to Cyprus, reuniting a family and enabling a young boy to receive medical treatment. Palestinian activist Musheir El-Farra described the experience: "For the first time in my life, I went to Gaza without being humiliated, without having to ask Israel for permission. We did it. We finally did it."

This moment was historic. It was the first time in four decades that ships had broken the blockade to dock at Port of Gaza, and for the first time in 60 years Palestinians could leave and enter their land, bypassing Israeli walls and checkpoints. Israel justifies the blockade as necessary to prevent the smuggling of weapons. According to data from the Israeli human rights group B'Tsalem and the

United Nations, the Israeli–Palestinian conflict claimed nearly 15,000 lives between 1987 and 2023, 87 percent of them Palestinian.

Although the Free Gaza Movement successfully sailed five times into Gaza, subsequent flotillas were forcibly stopped by the Israeli navy. Activists were often injured, interrogated, imprisoned, or deported, and their ships were confiscated. A particularly severe incident occurred during the ninth flotilla in May 2010 when Israeli operatives attacked the boats, killing ten activists and wounding over 50 more.

Despite the violent setbacks, the resolve to end the blockade and ensure a dignified existence for Palestinians continues. As of June 2024, the Freedom Flotilla Coalition announced a new mission dedicated to the children of Gaza, currently facing an unprecedented humanitarian crisis. The United Nations Office for the Coordination of Humanitarian Affairs (OCHA) reports that since the October 7 Hamas attack, the Israeli retaliation has killed over 40,000 and displaced 1.7 million people, with 85 percent of Gaza's population affected and 1.1 million facing catastrophic food insecurity. On January 26, 2024, the International Court of Justice (ICJ) demanded interim measures to protect the people of Gaza from genocide.

A growing tide of pirate care ...

These are three tales of pirate care, three uncompromising acts of grassroots solidarity that defy unjust laws and norms. They use and hack the tools, knowledges, and resources available to sustain the life of those to whom care is denied under an uncaring Empire. This book is about such people whose practices defy resignation and cynicism, and about getting more pirates to join them. However, pirate care isn't just about heroes with superpowers commanding boats, hacking systems, or transmuting revolution into poetry and back again. It is also about the everyday defiance of nurses, cooks, friends, programmers, amateurs, tinkerers, librarians, professionals, custodians, and kin who join together to practice care dangerously.

The trajectory of these practices is revolutionary. In addition to providing care where it is most needed, and in addition to refusing artificial borders imposed by Empire, they show that the world does not need to be this way and they prefigure alternatives. Practices shared in these pages represent an emerging tendency of today's radical struggles, hidden in plain sight: an archipelago of self-governing initiatives, collectives, and coalitions operating within, outside, and across Empire's enclosures and institutions. This book aims to help pirate carers recognize themselves in their diversity and band together into a federation of mutually sustaining struggles that can turn the tide against an uncaring Empire.

Empire was born in colonialism, slavery, and enclosure and matured into an unequal and exploitative system of nation-states. The twenty-first-century global Empire emerges out of the withering-away of twentieth-century socialist, anti-colonial, and non-aligned revolutionary worldmaking projects.[2] It reproduces itself through exclusions based on class, race, citizenship, gender, and ability. It coalesces around ever-accelerating forces of capital and its hijacking of technologies that are wrecking the social and ecological conditions that make human and non-human lives livable and joyous.

But if Empire is back, then so is its enemy: the pirate. Pirate care is the revolutionary practice of the plebeian multitude against Empire. In potent yet not widely recognized ways, pirate carers are striking back from a position of deep asymmetry. In doing so, they are opening up a space of political possibility. By caring despite the laws and despite all odds, they immanently enact a different, insurgent world.

In this book, we will meet not only courageous activists on the high seas but also organizers taking back housing in gentrifying cities, hacker librarians liberating "intellectual property," trans collectives cooking up homemade hormones, and many more pirates, including many whose actions operate under the radar of the imperial armada, tinkering, conspiring, and colluding in a world of contradictions.

Their forms of solidarity, new and old, large and small, are important because they challenge traditional notions of care, offering alternative ways to address living needs, often in the service of people neglected by what we call the neoliberal capitalist Empire's "matrix of care." This matrix insists and enforces the enclosure of care by an oppressive triumvirate of the state, the market, and the family. It leaves untold millions to die if they do not obey its expectations or don't fit into its categories (citizen, worker, consumer, spouse, heir).

Empire's matrix of care is failing everyone except the most privileged, and this is plain for all to see. This is why it is important to distinguish pirate care from the care practices of far-right groups like conservative religious organizations, fascist organizations, and nationalist movements. These also engage in acts of care, but do so based on rigid boundaries of inclusion that reinforce existing forms of oppression. For instance, during the financial crisis in Greece, the fascist Golden Dawn party distributed aid exclusively to Greek citizens, using this as propaganda to reinforce racist prejudices against foreigners. Similarly, in the United States, certain Christian groups provide shelter and food to the homeless but often only on the condition that recipients participate in religious services or adhere to strict puritanical codes of behavior. The "prepper" movement organizes resources for an anticipated societal collapse, but with a patriarchal and militaristic mindset that fetishizes the survival of its select in-groups and has nothing to do with community care. In contrast, pirate care practices seek to expand the circle of care to all, often to non-humans as well.

... against the state, the market, and the family

In the last decade, commentators have begun to reflect on the systemic nature of abandonment and uncaring so characteristic of what we are calling Empire. Ruth Wilson Gilmore has called it a regime of "organized abandonment."[3] Dean Spade has analyzed ubiquitous "administrative violence."[4] Fred Moten and Stefano Harney similarly speak of widespread "enforced negligence" on the part of public-interest institutions, which, instead of supporting workers, weaponize professionalism as an alibi for neglect.[5]

Uncaring Empire does not simply ignore care. It seeks to monopolize it and divide it between the state, the market, and the family. In building care in defiance of all three, pirate care practices challenge this order fundamentally, demonstrating that another world of care is possible.

For some people in some countries the state, for a time, provided some forms of care. But today, in ways we will discover throughout this book, those forms of care are in crisis and have become weaponized by oppressive systems. Autonomously organized pirate care practices help us take a nuanced position *vis-à-vis* the problem of the role of the state, which has plagued the left for many generations. When these grassroots practices, for instance, make undocumented migrants legitimate subjects of care, they put pressure on public institutions to grant people needed resources and protection from legal and extralegal violence. Thus, citizen activists are refusing to be reduced to cheap substitutes for welfare provisions that should be accessible to all. Rather, they are exposing the public sector's contradictions, toxicities, and routinized mishaps, engaging state institutions while declining to normalize nationalistic logics and administrative harm.

Pirate care practices remind us that state-backed welfare services we take for granted today were inspired by or created as a response to collective care initiatives that were first set up illegally. The public healthcare system in England was modeled on miners' mutual aid societies. Yugoslavian partisans built a network of underground hospitals that would lay the foundations for the postwar universal healthcare. Feminist reproductive rights networks in Italy paved the way to legalize that branch of medical care. AIDS activists changed the legislation on trial medicines. Trade unions fought for an eight-hour working day and injury compensation in the name of workers' health and well-being. Freedom libraries in the US South prefigured the struggle for racial equality in education. In our current moment of the dismantling of state services and the erosion of rights, we must remember the repression these movements faced and the situations they negotiated.

While state welfare services have been hard-won victories of the working class, anti-fascist, anti-racist, feminist and disability movements, and left parties, they have historically been laboratories for authoritarian forms of care. In some cases, the state itself adopts policies that selectively provide welfare to reinforce exclusionary social benefits. Denmark, for example, has one of the best welfare systems but is ruthlessly exclusionary toward refugees and asylum seekers (although they make a mere 1 percent of all foreigners who are granted residence).[6] In Hungary, the far-right government of Viktor Orbán offers generous support to families who meet specific nationalist, patriarchal, and pro-natalist criteria. These practices are mirrored by reactionary groups that provide care where there is no existing or functional welfare state. In India, nationalist Hindu organizations offer social services to specific religious communities, using these efforts to consolidate political loyalty and propagate exclusionary ideologies. Mafias in Southern Italy and gangs in impoverished communities around the world provide protection and economic support to local communities but enforce loyalty through violence.

The crisis of the state's forms of care includes the decades-old battle of public sector care workers with the "zombification" of their institutions: healthcare, social housing, education, and unemployment benefits retain the facade of support, but their essence is eroded by managerial tactics and chronic underfunding. As the theorist Melinda Cooper observes, in the hidden wreckage of these institutions stands the family unit, and specifically women, who are now responsible for the burden of care that was once to be redistributed across the broader society, a redistribution that was once framed as a civilizational achievement and shared social wealth.[7]

Recent years have seen a new wave of strikes from care sector workers around the world (nurses, teachers, cleaners, and more). One message keeps resurfacing from these struggles: these workers are striving not merely for their own value, but to maintain or restore the quality of these public services. They often take actions to do so in defiance of politicians and their bosses: they frequently, in small and large ways, disobey their managers and the logic of neoliberal governance to do the job and serve the communities they care about. There is a silent movement of frontline care workers and street-level bureaucrats to bend, break, or overlook rules to benefit service users and mitigate the harm caused by classist, racist, sexist, or ableist policies.[8] It is in this context that pirate care can offer useful terminology for those acting politically from an impossible official capacity. It not only describes the explicit and courageous acts with which we began this chapter. It also encompasses these artful, everyday acts of solidarity within, against, and beyond Empire's matrix of care.

The second pillar of Empire's matrix of care is the market. The neoliberal revolution was forged out of the idea that the market offers an efficient alternative to the state's provision of care. But we must understand the market as having always been entangled with the logic of state governance and domination.

Today, the market is involved in care in a million ways. Care is widely seen as a massive growth area for capitalist investment. The privatization of state services has opened vast horizons for private profit, from care homes to hospitals, from prisons to deportation centers, from schools to therapy. But market-based care is failing everyone except the most privileged. A market logic, by definition, cannot guarantee that all are well cared for, as capital needs exclusionary mechanisms of scarcity in order to thrive (and offloading the unprofitable care onto the state and the family, especially women). High quality privatized health, elderly, or childcare services are usually prohibitively expensive, meaning the vast majority of those who need them have access only to inferior support, often from a burgeoning informal care economy.

Amid Empire's collapsing system of care, wellness and fitness industries are burgeoning. They appeal to consumers who have been taught that their health is a matter of their own personal investment, and they appeal to entrepreneurs who see it as a route to personal success in an uncertain world. These industries are rife with marketing scams that particularly target poor women and ensnare them in a debt cycle. The faith in the healing potential of their products is typically predicated on the persuasive powers of guru-like salespeople. These industries frequently pitch products that appropriate non-Western cultural practices and knowledges that are exoticized, de-contextualized, and whitewashed for global consumption. The message of care promoted in this context is often underpinned by a simplistic idea of nature as a source of purity and by appeals to unspecified ancient wisdoms, which often play off of and into fascistic ideas about gender, race, and the body. Other times, the new care entrepreneurialism embraces techno-solutionism, aiming to re-engineer the body with pharmaceuticals, training regimes, and monitoring devices in an eternal quest for optimization, steeped in a militaristic discourse of resilience and preparedness. Naomi Klein argues in her analysis of these industries that when care is privatized and made competitive, it inclines its adherents to distrust public services and to loathe the people who depend on them.[9]

Privatized care is also organized through humanitarian philanthropy as major corporations and rich individuals, enriched by tax cuts and tax evasion, increasingly sponsor research, public health, and global "development" through private foundations and similar entities. These have profoundly reshaped the third sector around the world by completely changing the funding landscape, with a shift away from state and agency funding that is guided by public policy, and toward project funding that is guided by the ideological preferences of the rich. A case in point would be the Bill and Melissa Gates Foundation as the second largest donor to the World Health Organization. The Gates's support of patents made them one of the most forceful opponents to a resolution that would have lifted private property rights for the COVID-19 vaccines, making their formula publicly available knowledge and allowing many countries in the Global South to fabricate their own vaccines.[10]

The final pillar of Empire's matrix of care is the family. As the state and the market constantly fail to provide adequate care for all, they remain confident that the family will pick up the pieces "for free."

To understand this, we need to start from the issue of what family stands in for: a nexus between blood relations and a set of reciprocal obligations. Authoritarian care practices promoted by far-right groups are deeply intertwined with patriarchal norms. These groups often advocate that care be performed by women within the private sphere, reinforcing expectations that confine women to domestic roles. For example, in traditionalist Catholic and Evangelical circles, women are celebrated as divinely ordained homemakers and caregivers. The "tradwife" trend on social media and similar fads glorify a return to what are imagined to be "natural" gender roles, where women are expected to focus solely on home and family, relinquishing public or professional life. "Nature" here is an ideological construct, either a religiously mandated reality or a pseudo-scientific order of things, and it is invoked to normalize two sets of expectations. First, that we owe an unquestionable loyalty and responsibility to those with whom we happen to share genetic lineage, ethnicity, or nation, over and above those with whom we share other kinds of bonds—for example, those based on friendship, comradeship, or other elective affinities. Second, the family, posited as the primary site of care, naturally arranges people into hierarchies that govern the distribution of care labor, power, and responsibility.

Within these hierarchies, women's supposedly "natural" inclination toward care makes them subject to oppression and exploitation. Feminist scholars such as Leopoldina Fortunati and Amalia Perez Orozco have taught us that under patriarchal family care, labor is subjected to a double invisibilization.[11] First, it is a common drudgery that is not recognized as labor at all, but part of a "natural" relational life of women (three-quarters of all unpaid care work globally is done by women and girls, and women make up two-thirds of the care workforce).[12] Second, this care work is relegated to the "private" sphere and hence disqualified from being discussed publicly as a political and economic matter, even though a recent report estimated women's unpaid labor to be worth "at least $10.8 trillion annually," equating to "more than three times the size of the world's tech industry."[13]

Feminist activists and scholars such as Silvia Federici, Mariarosa dalla Costa, and Maria Mies repeatedly called into question the split between private and public spheres as the foundational error of Western liberal politics and economics, and have pointed to the gendering of domestic care labor as a key dimension of the struggle against capitalism.[14] This struggle takes place at the intersection of the material and the relational: the family is not only an economic unit but one at the core of our political feelings. As Jules Joanne Gleeson and Elle O'Rourke put it:

> Rather than merely destructive, capitalism is simultaneously productive of affects, attachments, fierce passions, commitments, and hatreds. Each of these passions provides sources of legitimacy and social assent for the continued organization of production and exploitation.[15]

Desires for intimacy, recognition, and belonging are disciplined via the moral economy of the family. In a world of debt, financialization, and austerity, the family bond is also more and more significant as a financial bond. In this context, a radical politics of solidarity must be attentive to the norms that script our passions and emotions, and must invite the development of "new forms for nurture beyond the family,"[16] forms of inventive transgression that can amplify and lend materiality to different forms of living together.

As we will explore later in this book, the three pillars of Empire's care matrix share the same poisoned root: private property. We know that the idea that an individual can "own" a part of the world, of the common wealth created by a society, and that they can be legally protected in their exclusive use and enjoyment of it (even when it has terrible consequences for others), is a very particular and dangerous aspect of the neocolonial system that today manifests as Empire. The capitalist market is fundamentally based on private property, and it has been so successful that today many things essential are privatized, from water to hospitals, from patented medicines to access to research. To enable this, the state must impose private property relations, creating a legal structure that enforces contracts or punishes those who defy this regime in the name of life and solidarity. Similarly, the patriarchal family, spread around the world by colonialism and at the center of the capitalist economy, is also based on the idea that the private sphere is the property of the patriarch, his sovereign space within which he may arrange labor, care, and affects as he wishes. Though the overt rule of men has weakened in some societies, and domestic violence is legally condemned, the deep structure of patriarchy, woven through with the logic of ownership, is still potent.

This is why the figure of the pirate carer is so crucial now to the rebellion against Empire: it defies its property regimes at all three levels. Pirates have always been enemies of the imperial property regime, not only because they raid and plunder, but because they refuse to be the property of the navies that conscript them. Meanwhile, the carer—as an archetype shared across figures such as the witch, the healer, the elder, the custodian— is motivated to transgress norms by the calling to offer solidarity and nurture as part of an entangled web of life, in defiance of the borders drawn by wealth, nation, or family.

Criminalization of solidarity

Empire has mobilized care as a terrain of enforcement and division. Under a regime of what sociologist Will Davies[17] has called punitive neoliberalism, public welfare provisions are cunningly reduced and reformed to perform policing and repressive functions. Caregivers are tasked by their bosses to report "illegal" claimants; surveillance technologies threaten to turn every clinic and school into a border station; and unemployment, healthcare, and other insurance institutions frequently penalize people for the effects that poverty or marginalization have on them. As Angela Mitropoulos observed, the neoliberal transformation of welfare into workfare breathes life into outdated poor laws that frame the poor as morally at fault for their suffering.[18] This toxic mutation of welfare infrastructures perpetuates discriminatory practices as they become more entrenched in bureaucratic and algorithmic processes, widening the gap between the "deserving" citizens and the unruly, undesirable, excluded "others."

Yet, contemporary discussions of the neoliberal "crisis of care" rarely center on the worldwide attacks on solidarity, mutual aid, and autonomous care initiatives.[19] In the twentieth century, societies legitimated themselves in part with reference to their inclusion of the excluded. Today, as Empire produces and then seeks to control "surplussed" populations (those dependent on capitalism for survival but not useful to that system as workers or consumers), the criminalization of care has reached a new threshold.[20]

Over recent years, simple acts of nourishing, protecting, and informing others have become increasingly criminalized. In Houston, Texas, activists from Food Not Bombs have been arrested for offering meals to the homeless; Spanish firefighters who risked their lives to save refugees from drowning have been put on trial; Italian librarians have faced suspension for refusing to ban children's books that tell stories of same-sex families and gender diversity.[21] The stories pile up, and it's not just individual acts that are under attack. Systems of solidarity and subsistence are being dismantled in ways that are less visible but no less harmful. Via Campesina, in their 2015 report *Seed Laws That Criminalise Farmers: Resistance and Fightback*, warned of how international laws are increasingly making it illegal for farmers to share seeds, severing the most fundamental of human connections—the exchange of sustenance. A 2018 study from Johns Hopkins University and the University of Essex, *The Criminalization of Healthcare*, outlines how healthcare professionals in conflict zones are being harassed, arrested, and prosecuted for offering medical care to those most in need. Amnesty International's 2020 *Punishing Compassion: Solidarity on Trial in Fortress Europe* offers further evidence, recounting harassment, legal threats, and courtroom battles faced by those who have helped refugees evade death by drowning or freezing at the fortified borders of Europe. These attacks erode existing forms of care and simultaneously render it difficult to emerge new kinds of organized actions. They operate through a mesh of institutions, actors, and logics, but the results are the same: an increased role of top-down rules (delivered through legal and moral parameters), embedded in algorithms and bureaucracies, and a concomitant system of surveillance and criminalization that works to threaten those who do not comply. This is the nightmare face of Empire's matrix of control, one where "care" is synonymous with the unaccountable exercise of power.

The criminalization of solidarity is not simply a matter of what gets adjudicated in trials. It acts on the level of public affect too. It takes the form of the subtle yet persistent pressure not to empathize with the wrong people, not to get involved in the injustices we see all around us. Such pressures often produce apathy, but they often produce vicious reactionary backlash cultures as well, where those needing care are targeted.

The practices of pirate care emerge specifically against this criminalization of solidarity and help people generate the courage to disobey. Overcoming the idea that "nothing can be done" is often accompanied by a willingness to break the rules to make sure those who need care receive it. Many pirate care initiatives disobey such rules conspicuously to draw attention to the injustice of the system and to reveal the forms of repression that have become normalized (normalized in the double sense of being enforced through norms and of being rendered so normal as to be unworthy of comment). In this sense, pirate care builds on a legacy of civil disobedience, but not to make a spectacle of transgression to shame the powerful. Rather, these practices disobey in order to show that it is possible to organize care for those to whom care is denied and intervene where care is no longer legal. In this, they imagine new ways of instituting care, starting from the compromised realities of our tangled relations under the punitive order of Empire.

Pirate care and pirate carers

Throughout our lives, we depend on the support of others to sustain ourselves—and the world in which we and future generations have to live. The rollback of reproductive rights, imposition of austerity, and criminalization of solidarity are all examples of how the relations of care are constantly being severed and rearranged to shore up nationalism, patriarchy, and value extraction. In this context, not letting others suffer and die is revolutionary. To stitch these relations of care in new ways that are not amenable to the state, the market, and the family is prefigurative of a world beyond Empire.

In this book, we propose pirate care not as a distinct definable protocol but a concept to help those already involved and those looking to get involved in defiant practices of solidarity find one another and discover a common vocabulary for what we are doing in a myriad of ways. Unlike those institutions of Empire's matrix of care, the strengths of pirate care are its multiplicity, plasticity, opacity, and capacity to adapt to local conditions, contexts, and opportunities.

Still, we contend that organized acts of disobedient care constitute a political formation that is more than the sum of its constituent parts. We join many radical thinkers in insisting that social and ecological reproduction will be the crucial theater of struggles to come. Pirate care is a frame within which to observe corresponding forms of militancy and to make new alliances. By federating together various forms of disobedient care, we can build our capacity to break free of Empire's failing care regimes and grow autonomy in social and ecological reproduction, creating a virtuous circle that fosters new insurrections. Our understanding of federation is inspired by anarchist ideas of alliances between decentralized and non-hierarchical groups from which no one is excluded, as well as the examples of democratic confederalism in Kurdish Rojava and in Zapatista territories.[22] We understand the act of federation as starting from different realities we inhabit to come together in order to overcome the shared structural conditions of Empire that undermine the collective human and non-human survival, thereby creating different trajectories into a liberated world.

This vision requires different ideals and models than the ones we often associate with radicalism. As many of the stories in this book relate, pirate care practices have a way of asking more of who we are, and on whom and on what we depend. Pirate care, as a radically feminist proposition, is an ecology of practices where the figure of the carer is also the cared-for, and where interdependence is a core tenet.

Many of the contemporary militant imaginaries on the left are still animated by the ideal of the heroic combatant on the barricade. But in contrast to the images of exuberant, youthful radical militancy we inherit from the 1960s and 1970s, with its optimism, joy, and rage, pirate care unfolds in a more melancholic ambiance, one marked by exhaustion, anxiety, and depression, and one where we must admit our dependence on oppressive systems. Thus, in this book, seeking out other predecessors, we have turned to the legacy of two defiant archetypes: the pirate and the carer.

Pirate carers are hybrid militant figures. They reconcile the virile heroism of working-class militants with the consistency of feminists sustaining community organizing. Their affective politics finds its nourishment both from spontaneity and organization, from the boredom of cleaning toilets to the thrills of delivering a rousing public speech, categorically refusing these (gendered) divisions of labor. Pirate carers often tell stories of their politicization starting from a moment of transgression in the face of an unbearable injustice stemming from institutionalized negligence and harm. Pirate carers give themselves permission to be in the world otherwise, to appropriate and share knowledges, tools, and techniques needed for their task, even if these must be stolen from the master's house. As pirates they recognize that they always navigate the enemy's waters with extemporaneous maps. The stultifying ethics of the professionalized care industries—codes of behavior like medical deontology or corporate responsibility—keep us locked in a moral cage, where prescriptions of "good" and "right" serve to maintain oppressive structures unchecked. Instead, we embrace a pragmatics of pirate carers: those who work in the messy, queer, and radical spaces where care grows not from compliance to protocols, but from tender, rebellious acts of collective survival.

According to anthropologist David Graeber, pirates of the Golden Age (roughly 1650–1730) and after can be credited with creating the most militant form of transcultural plebeian literature.[23] They created myths about themselves and their adventures to inspire terror and awe among the imperial upper classes, but also to keep open a space for the imagination. In word and deed, pirates were living legends of how societies could be organized otherwise at a time when European empires were expanding their project of plunder and enslavement around the globe. Most pirates were proletarian sailors who mutinied or enslaved people who liberated themselves. They were known to include women and people of no gender who escaped punitive societies. Pirates often formed renegade communities that were monstrous to their enemies, rebelling against empires and experimenting with radical care among themselves.

If the pirate was the nightmare of those empires, then the contemporary pirate carer can likewise be seen emerging as today's Empire begins to crumble under the weight of its own violent contradictions. In claiming ourselves as the descendants of pirates, we don't want to romanticize them: to use them not as moral, but as political inspirations. In the name of their survival and enrichment, pirates of the Golden Age sometimes contributed to imperial systems of colonialism, slavery, and patriarchy. But we want to focus on their attempts to live, love, and survive outside the confines of imperial control, insisting on a life against a regime of death-for-profit.

In invoking the pirates, we do not want to hold them up as heroes to emulate, but as predecessors of our lineage of mutiny. For people like the authors of this book (who are spared the violence of racialization, who have European passports, who do not live in poverty or in constant fear), pirates, partisans, plebs, freaks are the opaque figures that give us repertoire to build our own strategies of mutiny and betrayal. Their persistence in refusing to be put to work by Empire, striving not to perpetrate the same violence out of which they were constituted, is one and the same with their capacity to imaginatively open up spaces subtracted from the imperial logic. As one of our favorite bad teachers, Antonio Negri, taught us, Empire under which we live today is also a totalitarian project for putting everyone to work in the service of our own misery and destruction. Against its compounded physical brutality and bureaucratic coercion, we must learn new ways of making pirates out of ourselves in defiance of the state, the market, and the family.

We claim pirates as our predecessors not (only) as swashbuckling renegades but tinkerers with autonomous self-organization who offer us another way to see the history of care as an insurgent act. Their ingenuity, deceptive play, and self-authorization is our inspiration. No existing institution will encourage or license us to care defiantly or tell us how: like pirates we must give ourselves permission to care. To care earnestly about something or someone, under present conditions, might often mean that we don't have the luxury of being earnest about how we go about it. Like those pirates of old, we may use deception, myth, and rumor as our most valuable tools. As we hope the stories in this book show, today's caring pirates demonstrate an ingenuity that is fundamentally opposed to the ingenuity associated with self-interested entrepreneurship, which is one of the most promoted and celebrated values in today's mainstream culture.

Since pirates are not immune from reproducing imperial violence, we need to embrace carers equally as our predecessors. We have never not been carers: care is the condition of life itself, including human life. Carers have always been taking matters into their own hands and trying to change the world. In recent times, carers from whom we trace our lineage come from autonomous feminist struggles, from women-centered community organizing, from Indigenous land protectors, from the Black fugitive craft of constructing a "homeplace," and from transgender and queer struggles.[24]

This lineage shows us that care is not an unqualified good. It is not always about hot tea and hugs. Like pirating, caring is ambivalent, and it can be coercive and violent.[25] Transfeminist Marxist theorists have worked extensively to show that social reproduction, with the work of care at its core, is a key terrain of struggle and therefore it should be a key dimension of our experiences of political militancy.

We need to activate the carer in the pirate, and vice versa. To be a pirate without also being a carer risks being co-opted into a regime of property, even as its enemy, opportunistically plundering the world as it is without building one that is different. To be a carer without also being a pirate risks having one's care held at ransom by Empire and channeled into the state, the market, or the family.

The stories in these pages are a glimpse into a global uprising of pirate carers, a force in the making, ready to claim its role in a radical, epoch-shifting revolution. The pirate carer is our political fabulation—a way of dreaming up practices that allow us to sever Empire's suffocating grip on our lives: the soul-sapping grind of labor, the empty promises of consumerism, the quiet despair of domestic life, the disillusionment of citizenship, and the ongoing terror of war. Pirate care practices are the foundation for a new kind of revolutionary becoming—one that immanently reclaims liberated forms of lives and communities from the wreckage of a collapsing system.

Our journey into pirate care

One is not born a pirate carer; it's not an identity. One becomes a pirate carer by refusing the impositions of artificially produced scarcity and the systemic denial of care. The swelling wave of pirate care emerges from a million ripples, anti-patriarchal, anti-racist, anti-colonial, anti-ableist, anti-capitalist, anti-fascist refusals of systemic conditions we all share. We, the writers of this book, also come from unique contexts and struggles.

Marcell and Tomislav have, over the last 20 years, contested the imposition of private property through copyright, drawing on their upbringing and experience in socialist Yugoslavia, where societal property was the norm. The privatizations of the 1990s had a devastating impact, prompting them to explore how digitized culture could prefigure the abolition of private property and collectivize the production of knowledge. In 2012, they created Memory of the World, a peer-to-peer pirate library maintained by amateur librarians federating their collections. Working with other pirate librarians across continents, especially India, the Americas, Australia, and Eastern Europe, they have been fostering a network of custodians who maintain alternative infrastructures for book sharing between millions of people.

Valeria Graziano's militant practice was profoundly shaped by the *operaismo* movement in her Mirafiori neighborhood in Torino, and the broader Italian context of *autonomia* (autonomous) and the ecosystem of *centri sociali* (social centers). After migrating to London, these influences guided her activism in addressing issues of precarity, coercive unpaid labor, workfare, mental health, racism, and gendered oppression. She was part of various militant collectives involved in radical pedagogy, institutional analysis, and participatory action research, as well as organizing strikes and direct actions.

In 2018, the three of us began collaborating, orienting our interests in disobedient librarianship and radical pedagogy toward questions of care organizing. On the one hand, we noticed that many such care practices were being criminalized and denied access to resources, including data, information, knowledge, and software. On the other, we observed that most were also developing their own situated forms of knowledge: systemic analyses, protocols, practical tips, etc. Inspired by crowdsourced online syllabi created by social justice movements, including #FergusonSyllabus and #StandingRockSyllabus, in late 2019 we assembled 15 allies to write a Pirate Care Syllabus, complete with its own free digital library of readings and resources, aimed at documenting disobedient care practices.

Starting from the Syllabus, we convened multiple gatherings, both in-person and online, where practitioners from different contexts exchanged their experiences, challenges, and strategies for disobedient care organizing. We conducted interviews, discussions, and workshops, often in informal

Valeria Graziano, Marcell Mars and Tomislav Medak

settings, where participants could speak candidly about the intricacies of their practices, without fear of judgment or suppression. Much of the knowledge came from direct conversations, but we also learned from rumors circulating through activist networks, community organizing groups, and mutual aid circles. Additionally, we drew from research on existing disobedient care initiatives, which we often discovered through our networks and not through formal academic citations. This method of gathering and sharing knowledges was itself an exercise of pirate care, giving attention to the ways knowledge circulates outside the boundaries of formal institutions.

As if on cue, just a week after we launched the Syllabus, COVID-19 transmuted into a pandemic, exposing the frailties of Empire's regime of care. The world has since been battered by a relentless wave of climate-fueled catastrophes such as massive floods in South Asia and a staggering food crisis in East Africa; wars in Syria, Ukraine, Yemen, Sudan, and Gaza; and a cost-of-living crisis across the world.

These interconnected disasters reveal the urgent need for novel forms of organizing care. We are convinced that pirate care practices defy despair by giving us the inspiration to imagine new forms of collective life. We wrote this book to help those of us who care, defiantly, to consider our conditions together. As we navigate the uncharted waters of this profound crisis of care, we take courage from the etymology of the verb "consider": to look at the stars together.

Beyond carewashing

As the COVID-19 pandemic swept the globe, disrupting business as usual, the notion of care swiftly ascended to the status of a buzzword. It seemed as though care was everywhere, endlessly echoed in the news. Care workers were celebrated by politicians and in the press (but rarely appropriately compensated). Corporations churned out advertisements promising that their products and services were care incarnate.

We are among many who fear that the dilution of the term may lead to a depletion of its critical potential and the emergence of "care fatigue." We are troubled by the fact that expressing "care" has become a mere form of obligatory virtue signaling in polite society. Rather than serving as a catalyst for a fundamental reexamination of Empire's institutions, the language of care increasingly runs the risk of reducing care to superficial "moral" or sentimental realms, where symbolic gestures of "togetherness" overshadow substantive action.

Nevertheless, we, like many feminist movements and thinkers, refuse to abandon the notion because it possesses the capacity to simultaneously express an *ethical orientation*, an *emotional sentiment*, and a *mode of labor*. It is also the term that care workers use, often with pride, in their quotidian settings of practice and struggle, preferring this world over more theoretical notions like social reproduction.

Because of these factors, recent years have seen a burgeoning critical literature on the politics of care. Throughout this book we will take up many of these books for help in understanding pirate care struggles but also to distinguish our approach, which focuses on how today's struggles are helping us see a horizon for care beyond the state, the market, and the family. One specific aspect of our approach is our insistence that the question of the politics of care is also the question of the autonomy of technology. Critical discourse of care is often inhibited by an unfortunate dichotomy that tends to place care in opposition to tools, techniques, and technologies, an approach stemming, in part, from simplistic patriarchal paradigms of the nineteenth and twentieth centuries. Care was viewed mainly as fluid and unquantifiable, an inherent aspect of affection and intimacy, while technology was associated with rationality, instrumentality, calculability, and systemic order. Care was relegated to the domestic realm, while technology was championed as a tool of unbridled productivity for the public world of commerce and civilization. One of the central contentions of this book is that the opposition between care and technology is misleading. Pirate care initiatives whose stories we tell in this book, use and misuse various technologies, appropriating and adapting them for the purposes of instituting care. This engagement with technology aligns closely with the anthropological understanding of care as a form of tinkering, as articulated by Annemarie Mol, Ingunn Moser, and Jeannette Pols.[26] The Oxford English Dictionary defines tinkering as an "attempt to repair or improve something in a casual or desultory way," but Mol and her co-authors understand tinkering as a fundamental component of "good care" practices within and outside of institutions, a mix of experimenting and improvising which has the capacity of "holding together that which does not necessarily hold together."[27]

Such tinkering sheds light on care as skilled labor, crucially involving the sharing of expertise and the production of knowledge. David Graeber defines caring work as that which is "aimed at maintaining or augmenting another person's freedom."[28] The ethics of pirate care emphasizes the need to resist extractive practices of our digital overlords and to reclaim or build our own tools and infrastructures to sustain complex organizational ambitions. If care and technology are seen as opposed, we are not imagining broadly enough.

Paying attention to technology in this way can help us overcome another unfortunate dichotomy that would lead us to frame our concerns about care either around those that focus on the exploitation and oppression of care workers (including unwaged care workers) or around those that focus on those who need (and are frequently denied) care. In our view, we have to do both. The necessity of recognizing care as labor must be accompanied by the invocation of tools, techniques, and expertise needed to be held in common to ensure that this labor is performed effectively, equitably, and sustainably. We need discussions of care that highlight the fight against Empire's regime of private property, particularly in the context of technical equipment, scientific expertise, and other knowledge required to support the flourishing of diverse care ecosystems.

But equally, the struggles to prevent the denial of care must pivot on an understanding and contestation of the privatization processes that are making care systems dysfunctional for the benefit of capitalist value extraction.

Navigating this book

This book is a pirate's map of an emerging archipelago of militant care practices that are rising from the wreckage left of Empire's failing institutional matrix. With such a map in hand, as incomplete as it is, we can chart courses through the worsening conditions we're unfortunately bound to face. As the social fabric continues to fray and the criminalization of care escalates, pirate carers are demonstrating the radical shifts in solidarity that will be crucial for survival and our ability to thrive together. Soon, we might all need to become pirate carers, or we risk becoming complicit in the destruction of the social and natural world. Understanding and learning from these carers isn't just about envisioning a better world; it's about preparing for the unavoidable struggles ahead.

This book introduces pirate care through five defining aspects: disobedient instituting, critical usership of tools, commoning of private property, pedagogies of partisan expertise, and queer kinning. Each chapter is woven with stories from past and present, all defiantly standing against patriarchy, racism, fascism, and capitalism. The stories we share use care as a form of mutiny, and as a compass for navigating the turbulent political landscape of our times. As a small collective rooted in the Northern Mediterranean, Western Balkans, and Central Europe, our perspectives in receiving and retelling these stories has been shaped by our cultural contexts, making our mapping situated and non-exhaustive. In writing about criminalized phenomena and illegal acts of disobedience, we adopted refusal ethics in our research, to ensure that we do not expose these communities of practice to any greater danger by sharing what they do.[29]

In the following pages, we won't provide an exhaustive analysis of each struggle we high-light, nor will we focus on their setbacks. Instead, we aim to sketch a political proposal by showing how diverse movements of pirate carers operate according to similar values and tactics. Some of the movements and initiatives we discuss may no longer exist in the same form, but we choose to speak of them as though they do because the legacy of care they leave behind is ongoing. Pirates, after all, have always been myth makers. Like pirates, these movements defy linearity, bending time and space to shape the future not through their perma-nence, but through their ability to inspire, disrupt, and create new possibilities out of the wreckage left by Empire.

The first chapter, "Breaking Their Laws to Repair Our Worlds," explores the centrality of dis-obedience, illegalism, and abolition in pirate care. We examine large-scale efforts like Sea-Watch alongside everyday acts of plebeian illegalisms born of institutional failure. We aim to show how these can be part of dismantling harmful systems

Valeria Graziano, Marcell Mars and Tomislav Medak

and creating spaces for self-determined care. We elaborate on the need to combine the figure of the pirate and the figure of the carer as archetypes for today's struggles that can help us see beyond the horizon of calling for the welfare state to be restored (where it existed) and imagine other care ecologies. Moving in this direction demands a dis-obedience inspired by the politics of abolition and deinstitutionalization.

In the second chapter, "Care-Hacking against the Techno-Health Armada," we expand on the need to see technology as a vital part of care, with a focus on the medical context. The privatiza-tion of essential tools has led to the degradation of healthcare, but pirate carers are creating a politics of critical usership that challenges these trends. Here, you'll meet DIY healthcare hackers, queer groups synthesizing hormones, and tinker-ers repairing medical tools on the periphery of the capitalist world.

The third chapter, "Pirating Imperial Property," shows how property regimes undermine our capacity to care for our communities and one another. Housing, food, healthcare, and education are all dominated by forms of property that have their roots in imperial conquest and the enclo-sure of the commons. Today's struggles to return water, seeds, medicines, software, and habitation to the commons challenge the very foundations of private property's stranglehold on care.

In the fourth chapter, "Learning Together under Fire," we explore how care gaps force insurrectionary communities to develop collec-tive, situated knowledge in real time. Pirate care initiatives enact radical pedagogies, mobilizing knowledge to make care possible where it otherwise wouldn't be. Meet the water protectors, shadow librarians, and communities of learners resisting the criminalization of learning.

The fifth chapter, "Organizing Mutiny to Mutualize Care," unpacks how care institutions assume the heteronormative family and the private household as their supplement. It posits that queering kinship and organizing intimate mutualities differently is a crucial aspect of militancy. Here, you'll find trans kinning initiatives, hackfeminist self-defense groups, and those bending family laws to create new forms of belonging.

In the conclusion, titled "Swearing an Oath," we reflect on the revolutionary potential of pirate care as a prefigurative force already disrupting the oppressive state, market, and family triad. Through subversive reconfigurations of care and property, pirate care suggests a way to rewrite the code of social reproduction, rooted in decentralized autonomy and radical interdependence. We envision a future where these scattered acts of solidarity could federate into a movement, where care becomes a practice of joyous mutual becoming. This book is an invitation to take action, recognizing the myriad opportunities within our everyday lives to organize material support and collectively resist the violent negligence embedded in our institutional landscape.

Breaking Their Laws to Repair Our Worlds

Illegalizing migration

The Mediterranean sea rescue that opened this book was bookended by two tragic shipwrecks. On October 3, 2013, a boat carrying over 500 migrants sank off Lampedusa, claiming 390 lives. Harrowing images of bodies added to the mounting death toll on this route, sparking an international outcry that pushed Italy to establish a rescue operation called Mare Nostrum. Mare Nostrum was successful, helping 150,000 migrants reach European shores. However, its success led to its downfall: Italy ended the operation, citing a lack of solidarity from other EU states. In November 2014, it was replaced by Operation Triton, run by Frontex, the European Union's border agency.

In 2014–15, converging civil wars in Libya, Syria, and Iraq led over a million refugees to attempt crossing the Mediterranean and the Balkans. Seeing the horrors, activist groups launched search and rescue efforts on land and sea. Within a year, Migrant Offshore Aid Station, Médecins Sans Frontières, Sea-Watch, S.O.S. Méditerranée, and Jugend Rettet set up teams, ships, and planes to detect boats in distress and assist Italian and EU coastguard missions in bringing migrants to safety. By early 2016, with the political backlash over the "migrant crisis" and opposition from many EU states to accept more refugees, the EU ended its programs. Instead, they opted to externalize migration control through agreements with violent regimes in Turkey and Libya who passed draconian laws to prevent migrants from leaving their borders. Civilian search initiatives continued rescuing shipwrecked migrants. In May 2016, *Sea-Watch 2* was first explicitly instructed by Frontex to take on board the rescued.

Since WWII, Western European countries have adjusted their migration regimes to benefit their economies. After the war, foreign workers from European peripheries and overseas (post-)colonies were welcomed to replace those who were injured or killed in the conflict. However, the 1970s Oil Shock, rampant inflation, and stalling growth led to rising unemployment and stagnant wages. Liberal migration policies shifted to stricter quotas and restrictions, pushing migrants into informal, precarious work. The Yugoslav wars of the 1990s renewed the support for asylum mechanisms, but this reinforced a distinction between refugees seen as deserving sympathy and economic migrants viewed with suspicion. The arrival of migrants tied to the "War on Terror" and the 2008 Great Recession further heightened these tensions.

From a broader historical perspective, racial capitalist empires have long thrived by managing displacement and migration.[30] Enclosures, settler colonialism, imperial wars, and environmental destruction have forced people to move, creating populations "surplussed" by capitalist systems.

Capitalism manages the very displacement it creates through borders, legal status, and systematic denial of care.

The bleak trajectory of "Fortress Europe" came full circle with another shipwreck. On June 14, 2023, an overcrowded boat with 750 migrants began taking on water off Greece. Investigative reports show the Greek coastguard stood by and even attempted to tug the boat into international waters, causing it to capsize. Only 104 survived. Yet, a decade after the shipwreck of October 3, 2013, the international outcry was much more muted and no migration policies changed.

Outlawing rescue

The EU's shift to deterrence led Italy and Malta to deny port entry to civilian rescue ships carrying shipwrecked migrants. This escalated to outright criminalization when, in August 2017, Italian authorities impounded Jugend Rettet's *Iuventa*, charging its captain, Pia Klemp, with assisting illegal migration and threatening her with 20 years in prison. Nearly two years later, Carola Rackete was arrested for docking *Sea-Watch 3* in Lampedusa without authorization. Matteo Salvini labeled Rackete's actions an "act of war" and "piracy by an outlaw organization."

Similarly, across the Atlantic, the militarization of the US–Mexico border with the erection of walls, violent pushbacks, and vigilante killings, has increasingly forced migrants to seek remote routes. Dangerous crossings, such as a 30–80-mile stretch across the Arizona desert, often result in disorientation, loss of supplies, dehydration, injuries, and death. Under the Prevention Through Deterrence policy, over 10,000 people have died along the US border since the mid-1990s.[31]

No More Deaths, a coalition of community and faith groups, has been helping migrants survive these crossings since 2004. North of the border, volunteers leave water, food, socks, and blankets in the desert, conduct search and rescue operations, and assist those facing deportation. South of the border, they run a helpline and provide survival kits.[32] In 2018, volunteer Scott Warren was arrested for allegedly supplying food and water to two migrants in the western desert and was charged with "harboring aliens" (a jury found him not guilty). A year earlier, eight volunteers were charged with misdemeanors for providing aid. As migration activist Emina Bužinkić highlights, the current regime treats solidarity as smuggling "so that the logical and only next step is incarceration and punishment."[33]

In a world of Empire, political language is crafted to make murder seem respectable. Yet, the actions of No More Deaths, Sea-Watch, and similar groups remind us that a different narrative is possible. No one should be denied rescue, and everyone should have the right to safe passage. Against the injustices scripted by policies concocted in the remote centers of imperial power, the concrete actions of these activists challenge the logic of punitive neoliberal governance: disaster capitalism meets its opposite: disaster solidarity.[34] These militant organizations continue a legacy of civil disobedience, where activists put their bodies on the line to save others and reveal that the law masks systemic injustices. In a world where compassion can be criminalized, these groups cut through doublespeak, confronting structural violence directly. They take action where sanctioned protocols fail, and, in so doing, demonstrate the violence embedded in the dominant paradigm. They redistribute political risk, daring to create new possibilities for care and solidarity.

Care as piracy, piracy as care

In this sense, these care practices echo the forms of unlawful rebellion and renegade solidarity of the pirates of old. The figure of the pirate as a rebel against Empire has always been a charismatic one, especially for the left. However, rather than the hypermasculine ideal of a swashbuckler, we want to refocus attention on the pirate as a disabled worker (with the eye patch, hook hand, peg leg) cultivating rebellious forms of solidarity and care.

During the Golden Age of Piracy (1650–1730), the brutal conditions of "impressment, harsh discipline, poor provisions, long confinement, and wage arrears" drove thousands of sailors to become pirates.[35] Marcus Rediker notes that by turning to piracy and forging oaths of loyalty, these renegades waged "a struggle for life against socially organized death."[36] Sailing under the Jolly Roger, they developed mutualistic protocols that contrasted with the deathly systems of Empire. Booty was divided fairly, and cruel punishments were banned. On navy or commercial ships, injured workers were quickly disembarked, but on pirate ships, sick or injured pirates stayed with their crew and received medical care.[37] The doctor and his medicine chest were the most prized loot when pirates boarded vessels.[38]

Piracy is intimately tied to the expansion of the empires that the pirates' way of life sought to challenge. "Empire" and "pirate" share a common etymology, tracing back to the ancient Greek verb *peiran*, denoting attempts, risks, and trials.[39] On the one hand, European empires aspired to establish a system of exploitation and ownership over humans and natural resources based on the freedom of capitalists to trade and the (alleged) freedom of workers to sell their labor. On the other hand, pirates, uprooted from their communities of origin, exploited to their death, and dispossessed of everything, found in each other the courage to experiment with another kind of freedom that included direct forms of democracy and mutualism that resisted the emerging imperial capitalist matrix. The clash between these two paradigms of freedom persists to this day: one rooted in the state-sanctioned private property (over wealth, land, and the time and bodies of others), the other in bricolage practices of liberation. From positions that are deeply "asymmetric in relation to the empire," pirate carers hold open spaces where we can experience care as an abundant capacity and cultivate the arts of making each other freer.

In a context of capitalist supremacy, pirates of the Golden Age were vilified as the "enemies of all nations," a narrative propagated by European

Valeria Graziano, Marcell Mars and Tomislav Medak

powers, justifying extreme measures to suppress them and their forms of organizing and sustaining life outside and against the state, market, and family matrix. Though ships of this era may seem quaint now, they were at the time state-of-the-art assemblages of the latest military and commercial technology, built for unprecedented speed, stowage capacity, safety (at least for the officers and cargo), and violence, with workers integrated into this terrible machine as disposable cogs. When pirates seized a ship that would otherwise almost certainly have been their coffin, they were appropriating the pinnacle technology of their age and repurposing it as a tool for liberation. Therefore, it's no coincidence that those who used the printing press to disseminate knowledge, against the will of authorities, were also branded as pirates—challengers of the power structures that sought to control not just the seas, but the flow of ideas.

Like the pirates of the 1700s, the search and rescue "pirates" of the Central Mediterranean have built and repurposed robust technological infrastructures to provide care at sea. Sea-Watch operates a 14m speedboat *Aurora*, two reconnaissance planes, *Seabird 1* and *2*, and a 58m vessel, *Sea-Watch 5*, which can accommodate 500 passengers. Sea-Watch coordinates with Alarm Phone, a hotline alerting coast guards and civilian rescuers of migrants in distress, along with Médecins Sans Frontières and other activist groups working to prevent migrant deaths in the Mediterranean. This infrastructure relies on a large volunteer base and a small team of specialized professionals, including captains, engineers, medics, psychotherapists, mediators fluent in non-European languages, media experts, and advocates for migrants' rights, supported by thousands of contributors providing financial and other resources.

To sustain both crew and those rescued during long stays aboard the ship and stand offs in ports, Sea-Watch activists have developed practices and protocols of mutual support—technologies of care. By calling them "technologies," we want to advance an expanded notion of "technology" that encompasses a broad range of immaterial tools we create together—protocols, agreements, abstractions, figurations, and decision-making processes that enable cooperation, sustain life, and make freedom possible. These are technologies as vital as any machine.

In the (auto-)ethnographic account they developed for the Pirate Care Syllabus, Sea-Watch members Morana Miljanović and Christian Grodotzki highlight five protocols for care aboard ship: the buddy system of peer support between crew members; psychological support to the group before and after each mission; skill-sharing among the crew members; shared ship cleaning and maintenance; and a comprehensive agenda for caring for the rescued.[40] While the ship requires a clear division of responsibilities, Sea-Watch is also invested in breaking down the division between hosts (the crew) and guests (the rescued) by conducting daily meetings and "including guests in the searching for boats in distress with binoculars, in ship maintenance tasks and [in the] preparation of meals." Oppression operates in part by defining who is a caregiver and who is to be cared for. By dismantling these artificial divisions, those on board these rescue vessels turn these systems on their head and prefigure a different way of giving and taking care.

Illegalism in the everyday

In the last two decades, people facing precarity and injustice have increasingly had to devise ways to navigate systems that often seem designed to keep them down. Illegalism has become a daily necessity for survival. In the United Kingdom, like in many other countries, social benefit recipients are forced into the shadows, working illegally because the state's support is never enough to feed a family, yet losing those benefits would leave them even more destitute.[41] In Haiti, where electricity theft reached 54.6 percent in 2011, impoverished households have resorted to illicitly connecting to the grid just to keep their lights on.[42] In Serbia, families now misreport their living arrangements to qualify for housing assistance, a common tactic in a world where housing insecurity is growing. In Japan, over the past decade, an eerie trend has emerged: neglected elderly people committing small thefts, hoping to be sentenced to prison where they can find better living conditions and a sense of community.[43]

Any understanding of the new politics of pirate care must contend with the widespread phenomenon of "popular illegalisms."[44] Both pirate care and these everyday forms of making do are forms of political-economic protagonism against an

47

uncaring system and are rarely strategic choices but emergent responses to conditions. Both break laws, rules, and norms to defy a regime of death. Like these illegalist practices, pirate care is already happening, even if it doesn't name or understand itself as such. Such forms of resistance doesn't always come from self-conscious radicals but emerge from ordinary individuals pushing back against a system that leaves them no other choice. As Harsha Walia argues, migrants are, without necessarily being ideological about it, doing the most radical work in resisting borders simply by trying to live.[45] People involved in pirate care sometimes resist oppressive systems simply through their daily survival in ways that overlap, learn from, and even inspire popular illegalism. The difference is that pirate care practices are oriented toward a horizon of collective liberation and advance through solidarity, whereas many forms of popular illegalism are limited to the individual and perhaps their family or friends.

There is overwhelming evidence from both government data and independent studies that show fraud is a negligible burden on state welfare budgets, especially when juxtaposed against the colossal tax evasion of the rich.[46] Yet, the moral economy of punitive neoliberalism hinges on the concept of the deserving and the undeserving poor and the vicious suspicion it breeds. It serves to help convince property-owning and relatively less precarious workers that their interests lie with the rich and can be served by "pro-market" policies and tax cuts (that lead to the reduction of services), rather than with those the system has made poor, who just like them, struggle to survive under austerity. This has contributed to the dangerous rise of anti-establishment far-right political parties that mobilize around the threat of the welfare cheat and call for the strict and punitive promulgation or application of (unjust) laws to curb what they paint as widespread abuses.

Transgression is transformative

Thus, to become a pirate is frequently not a conscious strategy of seasoned militants, but rather a consequence of being compelled to transgress rules and laws that deny life. Such surreptitious forms of pirate care are already happening across many aspects of contemporary crisis-ridden societies. It is often the case that those who are illegalized, organize to support each other. Squatters support other squatters, welfare recipients help other welfare recipients, migrants help other migrants. However, as a true opening of another world beyond the contemporary imperial order, the political task is to transform that piracy into manifest, mutually sustaining, and federated forms of protagonism.

This defiance operates within and against the complex machinery of institutional procedures, drawing on past social movements and workers' struggles. Yet, pirate care initiatives differ in one significant respect from individualized acts of coping and traditional community-based care efforts. While these, too, respond to institutional neglect, pirate care does not merely aim to fill the void left by neoliberal cuts, nor to secure the immediate means of survival. Instead, pirate care initiatives craft antagonistic and concrete practices of care that implicitly (and sometimes explicitly) pose demands for institutional transformation: they act externally by embedding themselves as real alternatives to the scenes of institutionally sanctioned violence and neglect, and they sneak up internally by addressing care labor asymmetries and clamoring for radical institutional change.

In an era marked by accelerating ecological degradation, an ageing population, and the relentless grind of global economic competition, the crisis of care is poised to deepen. As the practices of pirate care will evolve, becoming more varied, potent, and undeniably revolutionary, they will also face increased criminalization, targeted as threats by systems resistant to change. Thus, it's not just that care needs to be at the core of revolutionary strategy today; it is imperative to understand that any struggle failing to take care seriously—failing to see that meaningful care will be hunted and potentially outlawed—is a struggle deluding itself.

Our challenge, then, is to further connect these acts as integral to a larger movement. In a nutshell, transformational care justice, in our times at least, is easier achieved by transgression than argumentation. Transgression is not only a reaction to unjust laws but a strategy to create a momentum of collective subjectivation—an awareness of the power we hold as a multitude of those subjected to various forms of illegalization.

But in the first instance, a critical mass of disobedient subjectivities can collectivize risk: the very root meaning of solidarity. A striking example of this is Planka.nu, an informal mutual insurance club set up in Stockholm and Göteborg to cover fines its members might incur if they are caught free riding on public transport. "Planka" denotes sliding through the metro turnstiles behind someone who has a valid ticket. In this way, riders avoid the cost of a monthly transit ticket, which is prohibitively expensive for many marginalized people.

This club is not just a way for people to pay less for a daily necessity. It is a very effective instrument in a larger campaign that explicitly demands fare-free public transportation, where workers and commuters are in charge. It is aimed at enrolling many people in a useful act of civil disobedience aimed at drawing attention to and toppling "the traffic power structure, where cities are built for cars" and public transit is an afterthought.[47] The campaign gained traction when Planka.nu militants revealed that urban freeways were being developed using funds originally destined for public transport improvements. Roads in cities are financed by tax money and are free to use, whereas public transportation is mostly financed by fares. In a system with progressive taxation, making public transport free is a mode of redistributing wealth, taking from the richest (who typically enjoy private vehicles) and giving to the common good. Furthermore, public transport systems like those in Sweden, where the ticketing and turnstile systems are electronic, have become a weapon in the police arsenal to surveil the population and target undocumented migrants and the poor.

By articulating disobedience as a political matter, Planka.nu are, like many pirate care practices, changing the very terms of the debate and issuing an unconditional demand that divides the political terrain into two clear sides: one can be either for everyone's right to transport or for a regime that prizes cars. Similarly, the rescue operations we have explored earlier in the chapter pose a choice too: are you for letting people drown, or for securing everyone a safe passage?

As Empire's matrix of care is increasingly policed, subjected to austerity and used to generate profits, it is all too easy to let opposition be satisfied with critique and perhaps calls for better policy. But these forms of opposition are largely performative. Pirate care practices such as those we have detailed here expand care and collectivize risk by transgressing laws, providing real and meaningful (and often lifesaving) forms of mutual aid and solidarity while also demonstrating, for all to see, the corruption and deception of the dominant (un) caring system.

Disobedient instituting of care

As we have discussed, today Empire's care regime is being weaponized. One result of austerity has been the excessive insistence that care workers conform to procedures, rules, and norms, compounded by the introduction of automated interfaces and other organizational strategies that remove decision-making power from front line care workers. In this context, care workers are frequently enlisted as enforcers of punitive laws.

For example, in 2017 England's National Health Service (NHS) passed a regulation requiring medical staff to conduct identity checks of patients requiring non-emergency care, a measure promulgated following changes to the Immigration Acts aimed at detecting and deterring illegal migrants by transforming society into a "hostile environment." In response, medical staff and patients across the NHS started the Docs Not Cops campaign, based on the principle that healthcare professionals are obliged to provide care universally to people in need. Entire medical teams refused to carry out ID checks. Many have also refused to charge migrants for medical services as this would place an undue cost onto those who are least able to pay and would normalize the idea that people should pay for care, which might soon be expanded to other patients and the whole population.[48]

On a similar terrain of struggles, the Greek Solidarity Clinic movement arose in response to the 2008 economic crisis that ravaged that country's welfare state. The crisis had left a quarter of the workforce jobless and a third of the population without medical insurance. In response, the first solidarity clinics were set up in 2011. By 2014, there were around 90 clinics and 90 pharmacies across Greece. They were located in squatted spaces or provided by municipalities or private citizens, and their operations were financed mainly by donations. Most clinics worked within a wider ecosystem of solidarity movements to address not only the health conditions but also the social and food insecurity of patients in an integrative way. Many clinics were run democratically by both medical professionals and non-specialized volunteers and operated on the radical principle of care as a commons, not only relying on the community for donations and volunteers, but reimagining the clinic as a focal point for reinventing life beyond capitalism. When the left-wing Syriza government assumed power in 2016 and introduced universal healthcare coverage, many of the clinics shifted to providing care to some 700,000 undocumented migrants who had come to reside in the country because of the so-called "migrant crisis" in Europe, discussed earlier.

Such insurgent practices harked back to the healthcare struggles of yesteryear. Famously, in the late 1960s, Chicago members of the women's liberation movement set up "Call Jane," an abortion counseling service that helped some 11,000 women obtain a safe abortion before pregnancy termination became legal nationwide.[49] At the time, women who could afford an illegal abortion had them carried out in unsanitary conditions, leading to infections, hysterectomies, and deaths. To end such practice, Jane Collective began to post up advertisements around the city or in the underground press, inviting women to call "Jane" at a listed phone number if they needed an abortion. Women who called were asked to leave their details and then were referred or clandestinely escorted to a secret location where they would receive an abortion under safe conditions.

When it was revealed that the abortionist with whom the Jane Collective was working was not a certified doctor, some members of the Collective came to realize that they themselves could develop the competence to carry out abortion procedures. In this and other ways, they managed to reduce the price of abortion from US$500 to US$100, and offer it for free to women who couldn't afford to pay, including many racialized women subjected to economic oppression. In 1972, seven members were arrested and charged with crimes that could mean a collective 110 years in prison, but the charges were dropped after the legalization of abortion in 1973. The example of the Jane Collective inspired radical reproductive health activists across the US to set up their own systems for abortion referrals, to write manuals for vaginal self-exams, and to strengthen women's reproductive autonomy against the conservative forces.[50]

Looking back at the whole gamut of practices we have discussed thus far, practices of disobedient care emerge as responses to the historical developments and crises of the capitalist state. The Jane Collective emerges out of the advances in women's rights and the growing import of the nuclear family in the reproduction of industrial capitalist societies after WWII. Docs Not Cops emerges out of the tough-on-migration politicking amid the continued need for legal and illegalized migrant workers. In these instances, care practitioners and social justice movements mobilize to provide care in contravention of political ordinances. Conversely, some practices of care are born out of disobedience and militancy, such as abortion clinics or solidarity clinics, while innovating integrative and commoning practices of care. Many welfare institutions became part of the public provision of care only after years of illegality, as hard-won victories by activists who were unafraid to break the law and social mores. Pirate care lays the foundation for such instituting for the future.

However, practices of disobedient care emerge equally as responses to the internal crises of care systems. In an era of neoliberal austerity, these systems are cash-strapped, and there is constant pressure to reduce costs and streamline services (where they aren't simply privatized). In this context, care systems are increasingly disaggregated into two streams: basic services aimed at the general population, and high-added-value services, aimed at a smaller population that can afford them or who have no choice but to pay a higher price to receive advanced care. High-added-value services can then be more easily privatized, while basic universal services can be more strictly managed and cut. This process of disaggregation leaves behind a zombified public care sector, with a workforce that is typically exhausted, and service users who resent its long wait times, impenetrable bureaucracy, and substandard care. Meanwhile, the burgeoning private care sector is able to attract money and invest in novel treatments, better experts, and more frontline carers even while generating record profits. This is the trajectory of many healthcare, elderly care, and childcare systems. The result is that those who can pay (or who are deemed worthy by a public funder) get to live longer, have a higher quality of life in their old age, or a better start in life.

The zombification of public services places care workers and activists at a difficult, contradictory crossroads, one that demands a response as multifaceted as the crisis itself. On the one hand, there is a desperate need to defend the remnants of public institutions of welfare. More than that, there is a need to uphold the very principle of public care as a radical concept, as a common, sustaining a regime of care that is not a commodity. At the same time, it's crucial to tell the stories of how many public care provisions have been turned into dysfunctional services, exposing the slow-motion robbery that has turned once-vital public institutions into profit centers for a few: defunded, staffed by underpaid and overworked staff, managed as enterprises, to the point of being unable to be entrusted with our lives. And beyond that, there's the urgency to call out the systemic violence of care itself as it currently functions— even in public hands. Care, after all, can be a mode of control, and dismantling harmful norms built into existing systems is just as essential as building new, liberatory forms of care. We need to acknowledge that even a fully funded public model can still be toxic, still deeply flawed. The future demands nothing less than a reimagining of care from the ground up.

The debate over entryism, reformism, or autonomy can only have meaning if viewed through the lens of the radical pragmatism practiced by pirate carers, whose disobedient practices are the real substance of resistance. Without this

vantage point, such discussions degenerate into
mere theoretical distractions, detached from the
living reality of struggle. Pirate carers—those
who refuse to wait for permission—remind us
that care itself can be an act of defiance. Some
of their gestures, once sanctioned by law, have
been cast into the realm of the illegal, as with
volunteers forbidden from feeding the homeless,
their compassion criminalized. Others emerge
from within social movements, where the urgency
of struggle sharpens, like activists organizing
mutual aid networks to provide aid in disaster
zones when governments do not show up. Then
there are the quiet rebels—teachers, ticket clerks,
social workers—who refuse to let their workplaces
be reduced to cold engines of cruelty, ordinary
people turned radical by the simple necessity of
helping, like doctors who resist performing immigration checks on their patients.

One of the most important features of the disobedient care practices we have observed is their
contestation of the imposed scarcity that has been
so pivotal to capitalism's reproduction. The state,
the market, and the family have always legitimated
themselves by pointing to a supposed scarcity for
resources, often a scarcity they themselves have
created by their appropriation of common wealth.
Pirate care practices, by contrast, demonstrate the
self-expanding capacity for care, which grows as
communities develop new ways of supporting each
other. This reconfiguration challenges the widespread notion that the "redistribution of wealth"
is the primary economic problem facing society. It
refocuses our priorities around the "redistribution

of care" that is, in fact, the source of wealth itself.
Pirate care practices, in their actions, imply that
there is sufficient food, housing, healthcare and
security for everyone and more, and that we could
provide these without depleting the planet.

Care-full abolition and deinstitutionalization

In an era when care has not only been attacked
and privatized but also weaponized, pirate care
manifests an ethic of collective dissent grounded
in abolitionist and deinstitutionalizing values. In
this context, "abolitionism," which emerged as a
transatlantic movement to abolish slavery, refers
to the systematic effort to dismantle carceral institutions that perpetuate oppression and discipline
via mechanisms of punishment. In addition to
showing how prisons and other total institutions
are a mechanism by which capitalism manages
surplussed populations and enforces racial and
class hierarchies, this movement calls for a fundamental rethinking of how society treats those who
do harm, rejecting mechanisms of behavioral surveillance, moral control, and profit. In political
terms, abolitionism emphasizes the need to erad-
icate institutional systems that police behaviors
and replace them with alternative structures that
support care. An abolitionist approach compels
us to ask: How are dominant care institutions not
merely inadequate, but complicit in the production of violence? Furthermore, how have they
claimed a monopoly over the meaning and organization of care, narrowing its possibilities? How

could we build alternative care institutions now as a means of withdrawing support from Empire's care matrix and also prefigure the world we want?

These principles echo those associated with "deinstitutionalization," a term coined in the 1970s in the dialogue between radical and patient-led psychiatric movements in Italy, France, the UK, North Africa, and South America. It signifies moving care provision away from total institutions, which are arranged to manage homogenized populations (aka the "sick," the "mad," the "disabled," the "old," the "addict") and that function to shut them away from the rest of society to preserve Empire's values of work, obedience, and normalcy. And it signifies moving away from the corresponding service model that structures care labor hierarchically around expertise. Deinstitutionalization promotes responsive approaches, where those impacted govern themselves and their institutions through deep democracy and collective self-management of resources.

This concept pairs with abolitionism to provide a framework for understanding the work pirate carers do to dismantle "total institutions" while simultaneously "inventing" new ones.[51] Abolitionism and deinstitutionalization, as intertwined traditions of both practical and theoretical interventions in care, foreground *repair* as a radical and transformative gesture, and as a way of exposing contradictions embedded in existing organizations. Repair, in this sense, is not some gentle alternative to conflict; it's a pragmatic confrontation with the violent carceral and hierarchical logics embedded within care institutions.

2
Care-Hacking against the Techno-Health Armada

We have argued that neoliberal care systems have disaggregated care services, creating a dual system of poor public services and glossy private practices. The increasing role of advanced technologies in medical research, diagnostics, and treatment has fueled this process, reducing access to healthcare for many while disenfranchising health workers from controlling the means of care. Despite rhetoric around "people-centered solutions," personalized care, and patient empowerment, contemporary care is being reorganized around technologically mediated processes that are mostly privately owned, streamlined and scripted by a series of pre-set black boxes, with fewer care workers having the access or knowledge to adapt them to needs and desires. This reflects a broader trend where technological development over recent decades has tended to deskill and fragment our collective agency as producers, users, and communicators.

For this reason, struggles over medical protocols and procedures have become crucial battlegrounds concerning broader political questions. Today, preventive, diagnostic, curative, and pharmacological technologies are deeply entwined with all aspects of well-being. They are central to our relations with our bodies, autonomy, and interdependence. Thus, we must move beyond the limited idea that care is primarily the inclination and labor to support others. Care has always been mediated by specialized technological means, and in non-exploitative societies, technology could be recognized for what it truly is: a set of tools for expanding our capacity to care.

Recall how the pirates of old used to seize ships or use printing presses to share knowledge—they were appropriating the key technologies of their day. Today, medical technologies are among the most crucial to our lives. Which technologies are developed or not, how they are made available or restricted, and whether they can be repaired are all profoundly consequential for human and ecological well-being. In this chapter, we consider how disobedient collectives and individuals in mutual aid and solidarity movements devise their own ethics for adapting tools, putting forth a politics of critical usership and rethinking the role of technology in care. In doing so, they embrace an early hacking ethos, confronting power imbalances in today's technological fields.[52]

A DIY medicine

The role of technological open knowledge and the ethos of do-it-yourself practices takes center stage in the work of the Four Thieves Vinegar Collective.[53] This anarchist group is resolutely committed to providing access to those who are deprived of medicines and medical technologies. They tirelessly strive to develop innovative DIY methods that sidestep the conventional barriers

Valeria Graziano, Marcell Mars and Tomislav Medak

hindering access to medicines and medical technologies. On their webpage, they state:

> The main three barriers are: price, legality, and lack of infrastructure/supply. Making medicines yourself renders these barriers largely moot. We want to empower everyone to seize the means of bodily autonomy and make right to repair for your body a reality.

Their achievements so far include synthesizing a range of pharmaceuticals, accomplished through the use of tools like the MicroLab V4.0, an automated jacketed chemical reactor that can be 3D printed and assembled with readily available hardware. Additionally, they leverage Chemhacktica, an innovative synthesis research toolkit that employs machine learning to uncover efficient drug reaction pathways, and the Apothecarium, a digital interface they have developed that further empowers users to devise recipes and assembly instructions for the MicroLab.

Using such tools, the Collective has successfully crafted medicines like Naloxone, vital for averting opiate overdoses, and Daraprim, a compound used for treating HIV-related infections. Their contributions also extend to the essential chemicals for pharmaceutical abortions—mifepristone and misoprostol. They've even developed Miso Cards, a discrete format for delivering misoprostol abortion medicines "printed" on innocuous cards that can be sent through the mail or delivered as bookmarks. Other projects underscore their technological inventiveness, including an Emergency Room Suite featuring an automated external defibrillator and the ingenious EpiPencil, an affordable alternative to patented and extortionately expensive (though life saving) EpiPens, which are used in emergencies to treat the potentially deadly anaphylactic shock that results from severe allergic reactions. Finally, their inventive Tooth Seal, containing nano silver fluoride particles, which boosts enamel remineralization properties and antibacterial efficacy against various dental cavity-causing organisms, offering relatively cheap protection to those who cannot afford regular dental care.

A fundamental principle of the Collective is that they do not engage in commercial transactions. Instead, they share their creations by extensively detailing the instructions online, allowing potentially anyone to replicate these tools, technologies, and products independently. Central to their ethos is the notion of DIY medicine, rooted in the belief that everyone should possess the agency to "govern their own chemistry." Although the public often associates with the initiative the founder, Michael Laufer, the Collective consists of volunteers hailing from diverse expertise and backgrounds including people and teams dedicated to biology, chemistry, data science, programming, and hardware.

DIY drug production has garnered a great deal of attention, especially in the media where it is often sensationalized. While some experts caution against independent drug production due to potential risks, others highlight successful examples of tailored medicines produced within hospitals and pharmacies as legitimate examples of a potential shift in the production cycle. Four Thieves openly acknowledge the risks of their technologies and actively work to mitigate them. They have been emphasizing harm reduction and safety in their research and development by pursuing synthesis pathways that minimize toxic reactions.

The group's efforts to liberate technical knowledge grapples with proprietary software and databases. At the start, Four Thieves wanted to find ways to make medicines without dangerous side effects. They got a big boost from a company called Chematica. This company had gathered hundreds of years' worth of research about how to make chemicals, and released software to help predict new ways to make useful stuff. With Chematica's knowledge and tools, Four Thieves managed to come up with simpler and safer ways to make important medicines. But then in 2017 the pharmaceutical giant Merck bought Chematica and re-released it as Synthia, and Four Thieves lost access to the software and the research they were using. Still, they didn't give up. They made their own version of the software and started collecting their own data. It wasn't as fancy as Chematica's, but it gets the job done.

The challenge now is to share the information and materials with those in need. They're developing BioTorrent, a decentralized platform inspired by BitTorrent for peer-to-peer sharing. Since cultures can propagate independently, one person can grow cultures and send some to another. Moreover, to avoid legal trouble or high costs, Four Thieves found that certain organisms, like fungi mycelia, can grow on book pages or CDs, allowing them to discreetly send these materials through regular mail without raising suspicion.

Regulatory agencies like the US Food and Drug Administration warn that making your own drugs can be risky. But Four Thieves believes that it's more important to help people who have no access to care. They argue that if someone is denied life saving medicine, it's a moral duty to find a way, even if it means challenging the usual rules and taking risks. In this way, the Four Thieves Vinegar Collective stands as a group of rebels trying to make medicine more accessible and empower people to take control of the technologies that make healing possible. While they operate in parallel to established medical practices, echoing the shift many hospitals have made toward producing their own medicines, they occupy the space of tension between expert knowledges, governance, and market enclosures of the means of production to politicize its many contradictions.

Carers as tinkerers

Despite the increased role of technologies in determining how we care, reflections from the field rarely tackle the issue head-on. Among activists and scholars of social reproduction there has been a tendency to separate questions of tools, techniques, and technology from questions of labor. Gone are the days when patients were passive recipients of aid, patiently awaiting the attention of medical professionals and caregivers. The world's most popular doctor, Google, answers

70,000 health-related questions per minute. There are over 500,000 mobile apps available in app stores that assist users to self-manage a wide range of health conditions. Commentators are now identifying "digital literacy" as one new "determinant of health."[54]

At precisely the time when the so-called wellness industry is booming, unregulated, and ripe for scams of all kinds, access to the knowledge of medical professionals, to treatments, and to diagnostic technologies remains elusive for the majority of people. In this respect, claiming that care needs to be reorganized around the principles of bodily self-determination and informed consent is not enough when this claim is detached from an engagement with the overarching political and social determinants of health that shape access to crucial choices. We need to uncompromisingly reclaim the technical as a political field. This means engaging with the knowledges and machines within our reach while bringing the question of the possibility of their partisan usership: can we tinker with them?

The figure of the carer as a tinkerer is indebted to feminist thought, particularly in how it reveals the continuum between the historical oppression of women and feminized subjects, Indigenous peoples, and the systemic exploitation of nature. Ecofeminism has long critiqued the interconnectedness of these forms of domination, providing a crucial foundation for our understanding of the entangled systems we seek to address.[55] Our approach also draws on the critical interventions of Shulamith Firestone, Donna Haraway, Sophie

Lewis, and xenofeminist thinkers who have challenged essentialist distinctions between nature and culture.[56]

However, unlike Haraway's cyborg, a hybrid of human and machine, whose interventions are often internal, the pirate carer as a tinkerer shifts the emphasis from the transformation of the individual body to the transformation of the social body as its point of departure. This shift is particularly significant when considering the historical association of tinkering with heroic masculinity, as exemplified by figures like Thomas Edison and Steve Jobs, long celebrated as the archetypical figures of social innovation.[57]

A powerful example of how the carer-as-tinkerer brings the concept of pirate care to life can be seen in the ways transfeminist individuals navigate and hack their access to healthcare, including producing their own hormones. Transfeminist tinkerer emerges as a potent force of political subjectivation, particularly in an era where the lines between the digital and physical worlds are increasingly blurred. These individuals are not only technically savvy but also very carefull as they reimagine the constructs of gender in our collective existence.

Queering tech for care

In the Catalonian mountains west of Barcelona, the GynePunk collective emerged within the unique setting of Calafou, a post-capitalist, eco-industrial community. Known for its innovative spaces, Calafou includes a woodworking studio, a foundry, and the Pechblenda Biotrans-lab hackerspace. Born from the observation that "transhackfeminists" weren't sufficiently empha-sizing the body, GynePunk passionately delves into the realms of queer activism, biohacking, and the maker movement.[58] With an unwavering commit-ment to autonomy and self-care, GynePunk crafts innovative, open-source hardware for self-diag-nosis. Among their notable innovations are the 3D-printed specula for self-administered Pap smears and an array of functional DIY lab equip-ment, ingeniously repurposed from discarded technological remnants, including hard-drive motors and webcams.[59]

The work of GynePunk is reminiscent of feminist self-help practices developed in the late 1960s and 1970s in the United States and which spread around the world. Many such initiatives focused on reproductive and sexual health, offering lay-led DIY gynecological exams, Pap smears, and procedures like "menstrual extraction" to relieve a painful period, pass it altogether or complete an early-term abortion. In feminist spaces of conver-sation, healing and knowledge production, such as *consultori* feminist consultation centers in Italy (which were at least initially self-managed), issues of health justice were typically inter-spliced with conversations around the politics of pleasure and tactics for self-care.

In 2015, GynePunk unveiled a biolab emergency box designed for DIY biohacking. This kit facilitates the analysis of various body fluids, including blood, urine, and vaginal secretions. The overarching vision is to create a comprehensive emergency gynecological tool kit. This kit has immense potential, not only for marginalized populations such as migrants who are denied access to health insurance or confined to refugee detention centers, but also for sex workers and non-binary persons, who are frequently discriminated against within healthcare services. Furthermore, members of the GynePunk community use the kit to run educational workshops, often hosted by cultural and art institutions.

In addition to these tangible innovations, the collective has ventured into the exploratory domain of the post-porn body performativity.[60] They've delved into reimagining sexual paradigms, drawing inspiration from Annie Sprinkle and Beth Stephens's ecosexual approach to "degenitalizing" sexuality and expanding sensuous and healing relations to ecosystems. They actively engage with the post-porn discourse and have organized workshops on "dildomancy." These workshops teach the creation of natural lubricants and the herbal treatment of vaginal conditions, reviving ancient West Indian herbal techniques that induce or support menstruation. In this respect, GynePunk presents an alternative blueprint for those seeking to reshape their social existence with an approachable and effective political praxis, grounded in hands-on improvisation and a transgression of received binaries such as traditional/modern medicine, productive/reproductive efforts, manufactured/organic matter, technical/political knowledge, and engineered/wild bodies.

Such ethos is clear from their online writings, zines, and interviews, where they asserted that they have blended these approaches with mechanical, synthetic, *in vitro*, and even biogenetic techniques to redefine themselves as an "insurrectionary socially-reproductive cyborg class." Paula Pin, a member of the collective, emphasizes that body-hacking empowers GynePunk members to perceive their own bodies as "a technology to be hacked," through methods ranging "from the established ideas of gender and sex, to exploring the capacity to start researching ourselves, to find our own ideas and technologies."[61] The other prominent member, Kinki Klau, emphasizes that gynecology and its technologies have to be decolonialized and points to the roots of that field of medicine in the brutal experiments conducted by "the father of modern gynecology," J. Marion Sims on enslaved Black teenagers, on the basis of which he developed modern treatments and instruments such as the speculum. Although its members have since moved on to work on other projects, the work and approach of the GynePunk collective helps us envision the terrain of struggles over reproductive labor (both physical and social) against the structures of capitalist production and their technological mediations.

Hormonal riots

Trans people are *de facto* or *de jure* criminalized in 37 countries around the world and are denied safe, legal, and affordable care in an even greater number of countries.[62] In many, testosterone hormone supplements are classified as a controlled substance and can only be obtained with a doctor's prescription. If there is no legal recognition for trans people, testosterone can only be prescribed as a therapy for hypogonadal cisgender people (that is, people who feel that their birth-assigned sex and gender match their gender identity). Therefore, so-called "gender dysphoria" (when people feel their birth-assigned sex does not match their gender identity) is not among the authorized conditions for using hormone-based medicines. Many transgender people are thus trapped in a paradox. On the one hand, the recent depathologization of gender dysphoria can be seen as a cultural and civil victory. On the other, it has left a definitional void that needs to be filled to guarantee access to medical care for everyone. In fact, this void pushes people who use hormones to do so "under the counter" because, for official healthcare systems, they are either non-existent or hyper-surveilled. Trans people, therefore, often advise and support each other via social media and other online channels to reduce the risks associated with purchasing and taking unauthorized hormones.

Since they aren't used for sport or war, estrogens lack the lucrative black market that testosterone has and are not as much in the spotlight. Open Source Estrogen (OSG), a project led by Mary Maggic, an artist based in Vienna, bridges citizen science and speculative design to develop DIY and DIWO protocols for "domestic" estrogen synthesis.[63] A parallel project, "Open Source Gendercodes," by Ryan Hammond, affiliated with Baltimore UnderGround Science Space, also explores the use of tobacco plants as hormone producers. By tweaking the plants' metabolic processes, Hammond aimed to turn them into testosterone factories. While OSG remains a speculative practice for now, Hammond's vision is more pragmatic and potentially scalable: creating a genetically modified plant that empowers queer, trans, and gender-exploring individuals to cultivate their personal hormones, bypassing the pharmaceutical industry.

These projects belong to a broader DIYbio movement which, drawing from ideals of collective action and mutual support, maintains shared spaces and platforms for pursuits like biology research, biohacking, biotinkering, and bioart. This movement is part of a broader tapestry of efforts to decentralize tools typically monopolized by industrial giants. Witness the grassroots efforts in fablabs (fabrication labs), repair shops, and maker spaces. DIYbio aspires to bring lucid transparency to the often opaque realms of science, democratizing the tools and knowledge that have traditionally been held within the guarded confines of labs. At its essence, this endeavor is a biotechnical revolt, aiming to demystify the way science operates, how it becomes politicized, and how its findings are presented to the public.

Typically, the corporate medical technology industry produces extremely expensive devices and processes that are intended to be used by highly specialized professionals in hierarchical and bureaucratic institutions and appear almost magical to those who receive care. By contrast, pirate care practices see care technology as part of the commons, as a project to be collaboratively developed, and as tools to help build and fortify different, liberatory care ecologies.

Maggic and Hammond's initiatives remain experimental, highlighting discrimination, and they encourage organizing around the alternative synthesis of estrogens. But the Fairy Wings Mutual Aid collective, a chapter of the US-based Boobs not Bombs project and an anarchist group advocating gender self-determination has produced a protocol for how to self-synthesize and organize the distribution of estrogen.[64] Estrogen is not a controlled substance in the US, so all the necessary components (estradiol, alcohol, propylene glycol, diethylene glycol monoethyl, and the lab and PPE equipment to concoct them) can be freely obtained. The protocol can produce 250 six-month dosages for around US$2,000.

Caring for the carers' tools

In the current trajectory of Empire's medicine, we're observing a drift toward a world where our very bodies form entangled relationships with myriad of technological artefacts—from the seemingly benign surgical meshes to the profound interventions of deep brain stimulators. This isn't just about wearables or devices that tether our biology to the vast digital nexus. It's a deeper fusion where the digital realm melds seamlessly with our biology, as with the under-the-skin insulin pumps aiding diabetics.

This pattern isn't just technological progress, but a reflection of a broader system in which top-down, unnegotiable protocols find new means to profoundly shape lives. High-fidelity digital tools, now pivotal in diagnosis, demonstrate this expanding influence. Data collection is part of health and wellness programs promoted by employers and insurance companies to save money. Workers are monitored via wearable devices and offered bonuses for behaviors deemed healthful.[65] The critical question here isn't just about who will take responsibility for ensuring this hybrid of human and machine remains humane—it's about recognizing that the entire system is designed to leave little room for individual refusal. As private medical and biotech corporations grow, they weave themselves into the very fabric of social life, making resistance not just difficult but, at times, impossible. We need more than personal vigilance—we need collective defiance, a rupture of the social fabric that these systems are built upon.

Instead of materially supporting care laborers, which would greatly improve the delivery of care, vast financial resources are channeled into the coffers of the major players in platform capitalism. Figures like Microsoft founder Bill Gates and former Google CEO Eric Schmidt have used their vast fortunes to try and revolutionize global health, but often in ways that present things like telehealth, remote services, and the associated investments in high-capacity communications infrastructure as inevitable advancements, deserving of substantial public investment. In this new landscape, techno-solutionist approaches are presented as seemingly benevolent interventions in civic life, masking the unsustainable and elitist nature of their impact.[66]

The machinery of care, while being central to the evolving structure of medical intervention since the 1970s, provokes an essential inquiry: Who guards the guardians? And under which principles? Consider the US, a titan not just economically but in its norm-setting capacities. The legislative architecture there hasn't adequately evolved to clearly demarcate responsibilities concerning the upkeep of technologies melded within our very flesh. This isn't just a trivial oversight; it's a gaping void that is bordering on perilous. It's one thing to have machines operating externally, but when we broach the topic of apparatuses like surgical automatons or intricate 3D body mappers, we're speaking of highly specialized realms. These domains require adept engineers and craftspeople, individuals not always accessible within the conventional hospital corridors. The burgeoning kinship between machine and body invites a profound reflection: How do we transpose the moral compass of caregiving onto these inanimate objects? Even a rudimentary tool like a defibrillator turns futile if compromised. Now, consider the implications of a faltering pacemaker—the stakes skyrocket exponentially. The quandary deepens when acknowledging manufacturers' penchant for monopolizing their technological marvels. They ensnare the process in red tape, stonewall third-party technicians, obfuscate diagnostics, and monopolistically clutch onto spare parts. While this might sound like arcane corporate maneuvering, the repercussions are starkly palpable for financially strained hospitals.

, Across much of the world, when a medical machine fails or becomes obsolete, it isn't simply a logistical setback—it's often a death sentence. According to the World Health Organization, in certain regions, up to 50–80 percent of medical equipment sits unused at any given time, not because it's unnecessary but because it's been allowed to fall into disrepair. This is more than just a problem of technology or finance; it's an ethical obscenity that requires urgent action. Yet, the very terrain where the hands-on diligence of repairers and healthcare workers intersects with the overarching welfare of society is fraught with contention, primarily stemming from the machinations of the corporations that hold property rights over the medical machines.

Against this backdrop, figures like Frank Weithoener in Tanzania stand out as unexpected rebels. Weithoener, an expert repairer in the field of biomedical machinery, redirected his growing frustration into "Frank's Hospital Workshop,"[67] a simple yet quietly subversive online repository of tech manuals and repair tutorials for common hospital equipment. This blog empowers technical staff, giving them the detailed knowledge to repair these devices—sometimes with makeshift solutions—bypassing the guesswork and reverse engineering necessary when hospitals can't afford official spare parts or certified technicians. Predictably, the corporate titans— General Electric, Johnson & Johnson, Philips, and the rest—responded with their usual hostility, wielding legal threats in an attempt to shut him down. Yet, these small, courageous initiatives have inspired a broader effort, with iFixit, an American company dedicated to helping people repair their technology, building a comprehensive resource for hospital equipment maintenance, challenging the deeply entrenched corporate control over healthcare.

Frank's diagnosis of the chronic maintenance crisis exposes a chronic underfunding of tech support, a lackluster commitment to preventive maintenance, and the neglect of ongoing training for those responsible for critical tools. This reflects a familiar pattern where "care work," which crucially includes routine operations such as maintenance, cleaning, and repairing equipment, though fundamental, is undervalued and relegated to the background. Stories such as Frank's Hospital Workshop offers a key insight: the concept of caregiving must extend beyond the human to include the care for the tools on which caregivers depend.

Radical critical usership

Pirate care practices, particularly those centered around healthcare, offer vital insights into our relationship with the technological realm. Technologies are not a metaphysical monolith. Conceiving of them as a singular technological apparatus whose instrumental rationality subsumes social processes does not help our political struggles. While the assumption that technologies are inherently bad should certainly be rejected, this does not imply that technologies are inherently good or even neutral either. We should rather begin by questioning what particular technologies do, how they are designed, to what end, and to what degree they are upskilling and empowering their users, and how they can be used, to what end, and how open they are to repurposing.

As we have seen throughout this chapter, pirate care initiatives often tinker with various technologies, adapting and manipulating them for their own purposes. Care for our bodies cannot be separated from concerns about our means and tools. Karl Marx pointed to the commodity as a chimerical object, a materialization of the exploited labor invested in its manufacture, and hence both corporeal and technical.[68] Class, too, is as McKenzie Wark argues, a "mash-up of flesh-tech."[69] The working class is composed of bodies that are the product of care work and also technological intervention and sustenance. Technology is not merely about tools or machines but rather the ongoing process of formalizing language through abstraction, a process that unfolds iteratively through feedback loops and becomes embedded in our practices. Success from a technological standpoint isn't measured by productivity or market value, but by how deeply these formalizations integrate into everyday life. When we understand a tool through its use, that understanding itself becomes a tool, feeding back into the iterative cycle of creation and reinvention. Feminist technology scholars like Judy Wajcman, Cynthia Cockburn, and Moya Bailey have highlighted how technology and gender are co-constructed through this very feedback.[70] Pirate care, in particular, operates from this standpoint by appropriating, hacking, and repurposing existing tools and systems. This approach is not about chasing a distant technological future but contending with the technological interventions that are already shaping our present. By tinkering with the present, we are prefiguring the future.

When we speak of technologies, we are actually often addressing a compounded object, one that includes knowledges and skills, but also affects and sensations, set protocols and organizational habits, laws and property relations. To engage one of these factors around a technology, to tinker with it in one way or another, often leads to an unraveling of other factors, too. In this spirit, hacking and tinkering within radical care practices do not necessarily begin as technical problems or solutions. Rather, they might emerge more like acts of critical, often collectively sustained usership that repurpose existing tools and detour their original ends.

We believe that pirate care practices give us the inspiration to confront the challenges of techno-solutionism that is dominating the way in which our quotidian tools are conceived and deployed. Radical critical usership, as a form of refusal, can be understood as an emergent mode of engagement, where individuals or collectives actively and critically interrogate, challenge, and redefine their roles as "users" within various systems, be they technological, social, or political. Instead of accepting prescribed functions, in which users are simultaneously "used" for imposed ends, those practicing radical critical usership actively resist, appropriate, repurpose, and sometimes subvert these technological systems to achieve transformative ends.

A radical rethinking of technology, one that positions it within the broader framework of social reproduction, is necessary if we are to escape Empire's enclosure of care, which confines our actions and dreams to the limits of the state, the market, and the family. But the queer, trans, feminist, and anti-colonial approaches we have outlined in this chapter also show us that we can no longer afford to imagine that our struggles over the fate of technology can exclude care. All too often, activism and rebellion against tech corporations, intellectual property, and ecologically disastrous consequences of capitalist-led technological development are framed as if they are struggles over ideas, economics, and resources. But they are, also, and perhaps more importantly, struggles over how we might reproduce life together. In this sense, the pirate carers' engagement with technologies is not only about repurposing and remediating existing technologies and their consequences. They also help us reimagine technologies and knowledges as a commons.

3

Pirating Imperial Property

Pirate care must be understood as an immanent act of rebellion against property. Recognizing care as labor is essential, but it must go hand in hand with challenging the ownership structures that restrict access to the tools, knowledge, and resources needed to undertake that labor and so to create and sustain diverse care ecosystems.

Property isn't just control over resources; it's the legally enforced power to exclude. It transforms abundance into scarcity, and forces a struggle for food, health, and shelter even in contexts that could provide for all. Under capital's grip, it extends across all aspects of life, from real estate to corporate infrastructure, severing the interconnections that sustain life. Those who own rarely have any obligation to even recognize (let alone atone for or remedy) the harm that is done to those who are denied access to the necessities of life by the property regime. The defiance of property is at the core of pirate care's fight against the privatization and marketization that render care systems dysfunctional. It opens up new possibilities for experiencing caring as a reciprocally freeing process.

Repairing healthcare

The recent COVID-19 crisis laid bare how deeply the ideology of private property is entrenched in the global healthcare system (and how pirate care initiatives can make a difference). Only a few governments, such as Spain and Ireland, dared to threaten to nationalize private hospitals and medical infrastructure in the face of the crisis, though these initiatives were soon called off. Most other countries capitulated to "market realities" and ended up paying astronomical fees to access medical supplies or facilities (the British government reportedly paying £300 per day for a single bed).

The stark contrast between the urgent need for care and the constraints imposed by the regime of private property became painfully clear in early 2020 when the Chiari Hospital in Brescia, Italy, ran out of valves for a resuscitation device used for urgent COVID-19 care. The manufacturer was unable to supply more due to high demand. A local 3D printing company was able to quickly produce a copy of the valve in less than six hours, offering a glimmer of hope. The manufacturer immediately threatened to sue both the company and the hospital for breaching patent laws. This was just a sad prelude to the scene that unfolded when even in the midst of a global pandemic, formulae for life saving COVID-19 vaccines were kept private, including the Oxford/AstraZeneca vaccine, whose development had been 97 percent publicly funded.[71] Most of the people on the planet, denied access to any vaccine protection from the virus, were the collateral damage of a global property regime.

The COVID-19 pandemic has been seen by many as a lost opportunity to revisit the role of private property in a global health system, where profit remains the primary driver of research and development. The Global Forum for Health Research still reports that only 10 percent of global health research dedicates its resources to maladies that account for a staggering 90 percent of all preventable deaths across the globe. Amid this bleak reality, the emerging Open Source Pharma movement offers a radical alternative, advocating for a pharmaceutical system modeled after the principles of open-source software. Driven by public health activists and researchers worldwide, this movement seeks to federate together projects aimed at creating open license drugs and vaccines to aid in the fight against dangerous zoonotic diseases such as malaria, Nipah virus, and COVID-19.

During the pandemic, mutual aid initiatives rapidly emerged as grassroots responses to the failures of state and corporate systems in addressing the immediate needs of communities. From local food distribution networks to neighborhood check-ins, these efforts were organized by individuals and collectives to provide care, resources, and solidarity outside of institutional structures. Books like *Mutual Aid*, *Pandemic Solidarity*, and *Social Movements and Politics during COVID-19*, explore how these spontaneous networks of support became lifelines, demonstrating the power of collective action in times of crisis.[72] However, these efforts were not without limits. The scale of the pandemic and the global reach of capitalism exposed the difficulty of sustaining mutual aid initiatives long-term. The reliance on unpaid labor,

the exhaustion of activists, the widespread illegalization of autonomous organizing highlighted the
fragility of these grassroots efforts, showing that
while mutual aid offers a glimpse of a world organized around care, it remains constrained by the
overarching imperial matrix. These experiences
remain especially fragile when they fail to escalate
the conflict by reclaiming private property or
establishing autonomous zones for the replen-
ishing of the tools, resources, and knowledge
essential to social reproduction. Without reclaiming these private assets, and a time freed from the
necessity of work, mutual aid risks being quickly
co-opted or crushed by the same structures it aims
to subvert. To transcend these limits, mutual aid
must go beyond localized responses and project
into a federative horizon—an interconnected
network capable of reclaiming resources and
creating autonomous spaces for care and solidarity that can endure.

Taking back what's taken from us

Housing, much like healthcare, is a contested
battleground where the forces of privatization
clash with the need for care. While in many societies today, single-family private dwellings are
often equated with safety, security, and comfort,
this is far from a universal experience. The very
concept of home, rooted in the colonial logic of
private property, reflects a model that excludes
many and fails to account for the diverse ways
people have historically organized living spaces.
In many cultures, communal living, intergen-

erational households, or collective housing are technologies of care that challenge the dominant paradigm of the single-family home. A decolonial perspective reminds us that the "home" as we know it is not neutral—it is a specific technology of care tied to capitalist, settler-colonial structures that many communities around the world resist, redefine, and reimagine. Yet, despite these alternatives, the single-family dwelling remains the predominant model across much of the globe today, shaping how we think about care and belonging. Still, this model is constantly threatened by market dynamics that view houses not as shelters, but as commodities, leaving even the most personal spaces vulnerable to exploitation and displacement.

In Spain, the last two decades have witnessed the rise of a large movement for housing rights—the Plataforma de Afectados por la Hipoteca (Platform for People Affected by Mortgages—PAH)—which forcefully rejected the toxic constraints of a marketized housing system, a reminder that when care is at odds with private property, disobedience becomes a necessity.

The roots of the PAH lie in Catalonia's long tradition of anarchism, characterized by collective ownership and communal living, with deep roots predating the Spanish Civil War. In the 2000s, easy credit fueled a housing boom in Spain, with exploitative mortgages and contracts boosting bank profits. After the 2008 crash, around 350,000 households faced eviction.[73] As unemployment soared and fees skyrocketed, many defaulted on their mortgages, leading banks to seize their homes. A harsh Spanish law allowed banks to hold debtors liable for the difference between the loan and the home's depreciated value, trapping former owners in debt even after repossession. Already before the crisis, the collective V de Vivienda emerged in Madrid and Barcelona in 2006, drawing public and media attention to the urgent issue of housing accessibility. Their demonstrations and neighborhood assemblies laid the groundwork for what would become the PAH, founded by anti-eviction activists in Barcelona in February 2009.

Over the next few years, the PAH mobilized debtors and allies to resist housing foreclosures on multiple fronts. It developed legal protocols to help debtors refuse arrears, forcing banks to renegotiate loans. It organized collective actions to prevent evictions, squatted homes seized by banks to help evictees move back in, reclaiming them as spaces of refuge and community support. It took banks to court, initiated legislative actions to stop foreclosures, and publicly shamed the financial players responsible for the crisis. By the mid-2010s, the PAH had prevented over 2,000 evictions and expanded to 200 federated branches nationwide.

Right from the beginning, the PAH organized via open assemblies, initially held every two weeks, where anyone could share their situation and seek assistance. They initiated weekly meetings for newcomers, a stream for those needing emotional support, and a stream for organizing actions and coordination. In all such meetings, everyone was expected to contribute to the organizational work

in rotating roles: convening meetings, record-
ing minutes, or helping clean up.[74] Many who
attended these assemblies initially arrived weighed
down by shame and frustration, belittled by
banks, the media, and the state as failures. But the
process was organized to help them regain agency
over their predicament and dignity through solidarity. The PAH created frameworks to explain
the extremely complex eviction process and help
people understand where they stood. This ensured
that each individual could identify their phase
and, during collective counseling sessions, receive
advice and emotional support from those who had
gone through similar experiences.[75]

A crucial decision in achieving greater organizational cohesion came in 2010 when the PAH
decided to gather signatures for a Popular Legislative Initiative (ILP) to force the Spanish parliament
to resolve the issue of insolvent families who lost
their homes and remained trapped in debt. The
ILP process provided a minimal reformist objec-
tive, but its clarity and justice garnered significant
support and built consensus within a growing,
diverse movement. The task of gathering as
many signatures as possible spurred the establish-
ment of coordinating assemblies at regional and
national levels. The ILP initiative was also accompanied by organizing *escraches* (public shamings)
in front of the homes of parliament members,
where citizens would gather to make noise and
make clear that each politician held responsibility
to support the ILP. After the right-wing Popular
Party (PP) rejected the ILP's text in favor of an

unsatisfactory reform of the existing mortgage law, the PAH agreed at a national level to revitalize an ongoing squatting campaign, known ironically as *Obra Social* (Social Work), mocking the "social impact" initiatives of bank-affiliated foundations. This campaign involved occupying buildings for PAH-affiliated families who had no other viable solution. During this phase, particular emphasis was placed on denouncing those entities that owned vacant properties and had been bailed out with public funds, notably SAREB, the "bad bank" established by the Spanish government to take on commercial banks' risky mortgages but run in anything but the public interest. The PAH's *Obra Social* housed more than 700 people.

What is interesting from a pirate care perspective is that in PAH we see parallel processes of political action, often staged independently and rooted in distinct political cultures, converge: open assemblies where participants learn self-organization; collective counseling and consciousness raising; reformist efforts to petition governments to change the law; and disobedient, illegal acts of squatting and reactivating utilities. Through its fierce campaigning at the onset of the crisis, the PAH played a key role in catalyzing the larger M15 anti-austerity movement in Spain, part of the broader Movement of the Squares, which began on May 15, 2011. That movement gave rise to municipalist electoral initiatives, most notably the successful Barcelona en Comú party, with PAH activist Ada Colau serving as mayor from 2015–23.

Living propertyless in this world

Securing a place to live has become one of the most urgent challenges in our rapidly urbanizing and privatizing world. Soaring housing costs shape life prospects, determining not only where we live but how we live—forcing many into insecurity, social exclusion, overwork, and declining health. For many, rent or mortgage payments exceed the troubling "overburden rate" of 40 percent of household income, hitting women with dependents, low-wage workers, and migrants hardest.

In many industrializing capitalist societies, housing for the masses was mostly rented or socialized until the mid twentieth century. However, the neoliberal shift in recent decades has drastically halted this trend. As real wages stagnated, public housing was privatized, and mortgages deregulated, pushing people to rely on inflated home values to manage loans and credit. Neoliberal governments introduced right-to-buy programs, promising to democratize asset ownership, but what they actually achieved was to entrench inequality and make homeownership the sole path to economic security. Rising home prices (benefiting banks and the wealthy) replaced social security, turning housing into the main way for the middle class to save for old age, disability, or education, replacing state-led collective risk management with private family assets.

The result has been a housing crisis of epic proportions. In the so-called "asset-owning democracy," housing values have skyrocketed, attracting speculative investment and making it nearly impossible for ordinary people to pay off loans. Life prospects are now tied to access to family wealth or inheritance, even for those earning a decent salary. Young people without intergenerational support and poor working people, many of them migrants, often spend over 50 percent of their wages on rent, living in substandard conditions, enduring long commutes, or facing isolation. A cruel paradox is that much housing remains empty, especially in cities, as homes are bought as investments rather than for living. These properties are parked wealth for the rich, supported by government policies that keep real estate prices high to maintain the illusion of economic stability. This perverse system funnels resources to investors and banks while doing nothing to address the housing crisis that leaves many without homes. Individualized homeownership fosters a particular moral economy. Those who managed to buy homes often reject affordable public housing: "If I had to struggle, why should I pay for someone else's?" This attitude entrenches fiscal conservatism, and as younger generations increasingly rely on family wealth transfers, it reinforces heteronormative family structures and conservative politics.[76]

The sanctity of private property becomes so ingrained that even in the midst of a housing crisis, squatting in empty flats is not only increasingly criminalized but seen as almost heretical. Populations readily accept the preposterous solution of outlawing homelessness. Viktor Orbán's government in Hungary, for instance, made homelessness illegal in 2018, forcing the homeless into shelters

or prisons, and legislated them out of sight. The
Hungarian activist network A Város Minden-
kié (The City For All), well versed since 2008 in
resisting anti-squatting and anti-Roma policies,
immediately rallied to provide legal aid to those
rendered unhoused, but options remain limited,
and the underlying issues persist.[77]

Housing infrastructures make us sick

The fight isn't just about debt; it's about challenging the notion that private property is the
main way to secure housing. Housing activists Iva
Marčetić and Ana Vilenica, in our Pirate Care
Syllabus, remind us that "the housing question can
be understood only in dialectical relation between
economy and grassroots struggles."[78] These struggles include squatting in abandoned buildings,
tenant collectives refusing to pay rent, and cre-
atively addressing landlord neglect or rising utility
costs. In all these cases, it is about people defying
the abstract rule of the market.

In the early 1970s, as Italy's economic crisis
worsened living conditions, the *autoriduzioni*
movement arose in opposition to the rising cost
of living and capitalism, by collectively agreeing
to pay less for a given good or service. Autore-
duction evolved from the earlier *autodeterminazione*
movement, where workers deliberately slowed
down their work rhythms. The first recorded
instance of autoreductions saw Fiat workers in
Turin refusing to pay increased transportation
fares. After initial success, in 1974, autoreduc-
tion practice spread to include electricity bills:

In Turin and nearby regions, 150,000 families managed to reduce their energy costs, supported by many electric company workers who refused to cut off power. The movement soon spread to other cities, targeting phone bills, heating, and rent payments. In parallel, houses where being reclaimed from speculation and occupied by families (in Rome alone, 5,000 occupations were recorded in 1974), with similar actions in major cities like Milan and Naples. During this period, the revolutionary left also began practicing "proletarian expropriations," where activists entered supermarkets and took groceries to redistribute. These actions revealed "the importance of the home as a unit of production,"[79] with housewives leading the struggle "for the re-appropriation of social wealth,"[80] and recasting domestic consumption as a terrain of struggle.

More recently in South Africa, the 2003 Operation Vulamanzi (Operation Water for All) also defied property regimes that constrain and squeeze value out of the domestic sphere by defying the privatization of water provisions introduced in the early 2000s despite the post-Apartheid South African constitution guaranteeing access to "sufficient" water to all. Households in Johannesburg's townships of Soweto and Orange Farm were placed on a meter and allocated a fixed monthly allowance of 6,000 liters of free water, leaving many large families cut off mid-month, *de facto* forcing them to pay for water at prices they could not afford or to haul water from areas that didn't have meters.[81] The situation hit poorer households hardest, as many included unregistered residents, who therefore would not be counted for in the official water allocation. The Anti-Privatization Forum and the Coalition Against Water Privatization, supported by radical plumbers and local residents, launched a campaign under the slogan "Destroy Meter, Enjoy Free Water." They systematically removed the meters and dumped them in front of government buildings and water company offices, returning the "private property" to its owners.

Afterlives of imperial property

Through rent strikes, squatting, and defying utility hikes, housing struggles contest the very premise that access to basic resources should be tethered to private ownership. This pushback against the commodification of life's essentials finds strong echoes in struggles over food and land, where the enduring legacy of imperial property still dictates much of how our world is organized.

The modern food system, where 30 percent of all food is wasted and 30 percent of the global population goes hungry, is a glaring indictment of that legacy. Modern proto-capitalism transferred land from a feudal hierarchy, where use rights were passed from the sovereign down to lords and then leased to peasants, into a tradable private property, transacted with money and governed by contracts enforced by the state. This shift helped to entrench an ideology of possessive individualism, where owning property became synonymous with a self-owning subjectivity, personal freedom, and political rights, at first only for ruling classes, colonialists, and then men (granting them a continued classist, racial, and patriarchal privilege).[82] By the sixteenth century, the European aristocracy and an emerging bourgeoisie had seized much of the land held in common by peasants for more profitable uses, like the production of wool and food for the market. This upheaval pushed peasants off their lands, stripping them of their means of subsistence and turning them into a landless proletariat, solidifying a capitalist, patriarchal system that would shape the centuries to come.

As European surplussed populations grew, economic and military competition between kingdoms intensified, and a new middle class emerged hungry for wealth and distinction, colonialism became a key "solution." This fueled the hyper-exploitation of colonies through the slave trade and plantations, which mass-produced stimulants like sugar, coffee, cocoa, and tobacco.[83] Recent scholarship in social ecology encourages us to see the systems that entangled humans in the broader web of life as a "social metabolism": European capitalist "modernity" advanced through massive biophysical subsidies provided by colonialism, the transatlantic slave trade, and other forms of imperial extraction. Private property, celebrated as the bedrock of individual liberty, was actually a tool of dispossession, destroying communities, habitats, species, and cultures.[84] Plantations epitomized this violent transformation of land and life into profit, laying the blueprint for global capitalism.[85] The legalized theft of people's lives and ecosystems, sanctioned and made permanent by private property during

imperial expansion, remains one of the most
enduring legacies of that era.

While slavery has been abolished *de jure*, the
contemporary food system still bears its colonial
imprint. One form of neo-imperial plunder is the
extraction and patenting of seeds and their properties. Among peasants and Indigenous peoples,
crop and medicinal seeds have long been part
of the shared commons, both as mutual aid and
as a way to increase genetic diversity against
disease and threats. It was understood that caring
for the land ensured care in return. Since the
1980s, with genetic engineering and seed patenting, agrichemical corporations like Monsanto,
Syngenta, and Dow have focused on developing
or discovering crops resistant to environmental
stress or pests, or with certain nutritive or medicinal benefits. Intellectual property laws secure
these companies' profits, give them control over
germplasm, and lock farmers into dependence on
their technologies, shaping the direction of development of food systems in both the Global North
and South.

Farmers are often forced to take on loans to buy
patented seeds annually, instead of getting them
naturally, and to grow cash crops for the global
market rather than local needs. When harvests fail
due to bad weather, price instability, or rising fer-
tilizer and energy costs—all common in today's
climate crisis and conflict-ridden era—farmers
are left with crippling debt. Many become inden-
tured to agribusiness and loan sharks, a pattern
long supported by the World Bank and IMF, which

push neoliberal policies favoring market-driven "development."

The transformation of plants' genetic code into private property has triggered waves of global protests, focusing on pesticides, GMOs, biodiversity loss, farmers' rights, and food sovereignty. Vandana Shiva has raised awareness of the harmful effects of seed patenting on subsistence farmers, Indigenous knowledge, and community resilience, urging activists to "occupy the seed" and fight for "seed freedom."[86] Seed banks and exchanges have been established worldwide to preserve and share non-proprietary seeds.

Some activists are tackling the problem at its root by preventing seed privatization altogether. One such approach is turning intellectual property against itself. The Open Source Seed Initiative (OSSI), founded in the US in 2011, aims to create a repository of plant varieties that cannot be patented. OSSI collaborates with plant breeders, farmers, and seed companies, ensuring that the varieties they develop remain freely available under four key freedoms: to grow, share, sell, and use the seeds for further breeding without restriction. These four freedoms mirror the GNU General Public License of the Free Software movement, which empowers developers to share their code and its outcomes, recognizing the collaborative nature of all culture and technology. Just as the "copyleft" in Free Software ensures no one can privatize code created from collective labor—a common—the OSSI pledge ensures that no one can "restrict others' use of these seeds or their derivatives by patents or other means."[87]

OSSI released its first unpatentable broccoli, kale, and celery seeds in 2014. A decade later, its repository holds 553 seed varieties available through OSSI's pledgers.

Intellectual property not only encloses the knowledge and genetic commons, it also encloses our ability to share, care for, and repair vital tools, just as we saw in the last chapter. For example, John Deere, an agricultural machinery giant, has been using embedded software and a licensing agreement to effectively prevent farmers from having their tractors repaired or modified by anyone other than John Deere's authorized repair partners.[88] Farming can be a time-critical operation, and malfunctioning equipment can spell doom for a farmer. As farms tend to be in remote, sometimes hard-to-reach places, authorized repair can arrive too late. Since 2016, John Deere's license agreement has effectively prohibited unauthorized repairs, forcing farmers to absolve the company of liability for crop loss, lost profits, goodwill, or equipment use resulting from any software issues. In retaliation, US farmers began buying cheap versions of John Deere firmware and passkey generators from Polish and Ukrainian hackers to crack their tractors' software. This lets them repair malfunctions and modify equipment, like running it on methane from pig manure.[89] These farmers have also become key players in the growing Right to Repair movement, advocating for the freedom to fix and improve the tools that sustain their livelihoods.

Repossessions

As we confront the intertwined crises of ecological collapse and an aging global population,
neoliberal governments will likely deepen
their dependence on market solutions, further
entrenching the privatization of our most essential common goods—housing, water, food, and
healthcare. This increasing reliance on private
property to manage the very fabric of our existence is both ethically and politically indefensible.

In this context, any struggle for a society
centered on care must fundamentally challenge
the concept of private property and commit to
a serious study of commoning: a commitment
to collective decision-making processes, diverse
forms of accountability, and reciprocity.

The commodification of social reproduction
and privatization of care have handed our lives
to profit-driven corporations, leaving care labor
fragmented and undervalued. The results are
clear: devaluing care and monopolizing resources
are two sides of the same system, reducing all life
forms to commodities. Figuring out how to reclaim
and redistribute what's been stolen through pirate
care practices creates spaces for the commons
to flourish and for different subjectivities to be
composed. Repossession is not just a tactic—it's a
declaration of care.

4
Learning Together under Fire

In April 2016, members of the Standing Rock Sioux Reservation and neighboring Native American communities established a camp at the confluence of the Missouri and Cannonball Rivers to block the Dakota Access Pipeline. This US$4 billion project, extending from the shale oil fields in North Dakota to Illinois, was planned to tunnel under the Missouri River and Lake Oahe reservoir—vital water sources for territories of the Great Sioux Reservation along their western shores. Since the project was announced in 2014, Sioux people, the Indigenous Environmental Network, and many others warned of potential ecological risks. Moreover, the project would disturb numerous burial and sacred sites along its 1,172-mile route and violate land rights guaranteed by the 1851 Treaty of Traverse des Sioux and the 1868 Treaty of Fort Laramie.

When construction machinery began clearing the way for the pipeline in 2016, water protectors from far and wide converged on the camp. On September 3, demonstrators entered a nearby construction zone to stop bulldozers from digging through a suspected sacred site. They were met by private security armed with batons, dogs, and pepper spray, leaving many protesters injured. This incident galvanized further support, with members of hundreds of Indigenous people and thousands of supporters joining the Sacred Stone Camp. To accommodate the growing numbers, water protectors set up another camp on the developer's private property, (re)claiming it as Native land. As winter approached, with temperatures dropping below −20C, they organized day-to-day life for the standoff: a field kitchen, renewable energy generators, meeting and ritual spaces, a makeshift school, recreational activities, and training for direct action and first aid.

In a system where private property is sacred, sabotaging private enterprise is criminalized, and blocking infrastructure is seen as a threat to the state, this couldn't be tolerated for long. On October 27, riot police, state troopers, and the National Guard cleared the camp using rubber bullets, concussion grenades, noise guns, mace, and pepper spray. This escalation led to weeks of riots, culminating in a historic clash in November. As the risk of fatalities grew, President Obama halted the project, though it was later reapproved and completed under the Trump administration.

As demonstrators fought against machinery and mace at the confluence of the Missouri and Cannonball rivers, supporters mobilized elsewhere. The NYC Stands with Standing Rock committee organized teach-ins and created a comprehensive syllabus to enlist more allies. Their collection of resources contextualized the events "in a broader historical, political, economic, and social context going back over 500 years to Columbus, the founding of the United States on slavery, private property, and dispossession, and the rise of global carbon supply and demand." The committee offered its syllabus as "a tool to access research usually kept behind paywalls," inviting people to "[s]hare, add, and discuss using the hashtag #StandingRockSyllabus on social media."[90]

Such collectively assembled learning materials and the associated pedagogies are a salient feature of the present-day insurrections. They provide rare occasions when our collective capacity to act and our capacity to learn come into alignment in defiance of the imperial order and its relentless push to turn knowledge into private property. The philosopher of science Isabelle Stengers has described such experimental, experiential, and specialized knowledge emerging from and inhering to a group's practice as a "common." This is a shared knowledge that makes a group "think, imagine, cooperate," and it stands in opposition to the obtuseness of technocratic expertise and governance.[91]

Mutualism in learning

The #StandingRockSyllabus is just one example of the growing phenomenon of #syllabi—crowdsourced, autonomously created, and maintained within social justice movements using available online tools. This trend dates back to August 2014, when Ferguson, Missouri, erupted in protests after the police murder of Michael Brown, a Black teenager. Amid the turmoil, Dr. Marcia Chatelain, a Georgetown University professor, urged educators to devote the first day of class to these horrific events and the uprising they sparked. Using the hashtag #FergusonSyllabus, she invited others to share resources, sparking widespread engagement beyond the classroom.

Around the same time, the internet was a battleground for another struggle. As the #Gamergate harassment campaign targeted women in the gaming industry, unleashing a torrent of misogyny, *The New Inquiry* editors created a "Gaming and Feminism" syllabus to offer readers curated background materials. This method of collective learning spread quickly. When Donald Trump announced his first presidential candidacy, his noxious rhetoric spurred the creation of "Trump 101," followed by "Trump Syllabus 2.0," and the "Rape Culture Syllabus." Soon after, the #PRSyllabus (in response to Puerto Rico's neocolonial debt crisis), #ImmigrationSyllabus (in response to Trump's immigration policies), and #WakandaSyllabus (in response to Marvel's Black Panther film) emerged, followed by many more.

The creation of the #syllabi within social movements pushes against violent scenarios as a practice of collective care for what radical pedagogy theorists call "really-useful knowledge," or knowledge that can be used to challenge oppression, as opposed to the supposedly "useful" knowledge that is routinely favored by corporate interests.[92]

In our own practice with the Pirate Care Syllabus, we aimed to create a learning resource that brings together pragmatic knowledge and situated analysis from diverse repressed care practices, ranging from housing struggles and transhackfeminism to peer-to-peer health support, migrant rescue missions, and digital piracy. Our wager has been that these practices can juxtapose themselves and connect, learning from antagonism to antagonism, transferring fire to fire, passing knowledge from militant to militant, to compose an ecosystem of federated mutualisms.

While inspired by #syllabi, we wanted to guard against their ephemerality. Since they rely on corporate social media platforms, their longevity is often uncertain, and because they are often created with the haste of an urgent moment, their creators don't always think in long-term ways about sustaining websites or databases. Many links in the #syllabi created over the past decade no longer work, or the material has disappeared behind paywalls. While #syllabi resemble other ephemeral social movement media like pamphlets, zines, and blogs, in the tradition of radical archivists, we strive to preserve these resources to maintain intergenerational connections between past experiences and contemporary struggles.

With the Pirate Care Syllabus, we worked together with a small crew of pirate care practitioners to digitize and preserve their educational tools in plaintext, HTML, and PDF formats (which have proved most resilient to digital decay) using a free software platform we built called *Sandpoints*. It might not last forever, but certainly longer than the self-made websites or social media platforms running on corporate server clouds. The majority of resources referenced in #syllabi were originally locked behind paywalls, including digital books, academic texts, and newspaper articles. To break down these barriers, we've embedded a digital library within the Pirate Care Syllabus on *Sandpoints*, offering all the referred-to documents, books, and articles for free in PDF format. Both the syllabus and the associated library can be downloaded as a static website to a USB drive to be used locally, whether in a prison, a remote encampment of water protectors, or anywhere else internet access is limited or surveilled.

We wanted to launch and enrich the Pirate Care Syllabus during a gathering we planned for 2020, a summer camp for pirate carers on an island, where people could learn together and expand the syllabus. But the arrival of the COVID-19 pandemic made that impossible. However, as the topics of care and disobedience became more important than ever, the Pirate Care Syllabus was autonomously picked up, used, and transformed by others in ways we could not have expected. It was a reminder that decentralized popular pedagogies have a life of their own and that while local realities may differ, people are oppressed by the same systemic forces.

How our common knowledge gets robbed . . .

Care is a complex, relational, and intentional set of practices that thrives on shared knowledge and collective wisdom. Yet, one way care work is devalued is through the myth that it is simple, unskilled, or instinctual. The knowledges that underpin our collective capacity to care are increasingly walled off, treated as property by capital. As seen in the patenting of seeds and the sabotage of the right to repair, intellectual property turns communal resources into private assets, restricting access to vital insights and tools. To care is to rebel against these enclosures and insist that knowledge is a common, as our survival depends on it. Against such backdrop, struggles over knowledge in all of its facets—who gets to learn what and how, under which conditions, and with what consequences and costs—are all essential dimensions of pirate care.

In September 2010, Aaron Swartz, a student at MIT, placed a laptop in a network maintenance closet to execute a script that downloaded the entire JSTOR repository, one of the world's largest paywalled collections of scientific texts. Five months later, he was apprehended by police and Secret Service agents and eventually charged with 13 felony counts, facing up to 50 years in prison and US$1 million in fines. Swartz, a gifted programmer who helped build Reddit and some of the internet's infrastructure, was a staunch advocate of universal access to knowledge. He had previously been known to federal prosecutors for releasing federal court documents, which, though public domain, were locked in paywalled databases. Tragically, under pressure to accept a lengthy prison sentence for liberating JSTOR's scientific knowledge, Swartz committed suicide on January 11, 2013. This came in the wake of the disclosure that he was the author of a 2008 *Guerilla Open Access Manifesto*, in which he wrote:

Information is power. But like all power, there are those who want to keep it for themselves.

The world's entire scientific and cultural heritage, published over centuries in books and journals, is increasingly being digitized and locked up by a handful of private corporations. Want to read the papers featuring the most famous results of the sciences? You'll need to send enormous amounts to publishers like Reed Elsevier . . . We need to take information, wherever it is stored, make our copies and share them with the world. We need to take stuff that's out of copyright and add it to the archive. We need to buy secret databases and put them on the Web. We need to download scientific journals and upload them to file sharing networks. We need to fight for Guerilla Open Access. With enough of us, around the world, we'll not just send a strong message opposing the privatization of knowledge—we'll make it a thing of the past. Will you join us?[93]

Swartz never denied responsibility for his acts but rather articulated them as civil disobedience against unjust laws. In the *Guerilla Open Access Manifesto* he framed the everyday practice of sharing books and articles, which has been the basis of the growth of knowledge, as the precedent for an ethical duty for political action against the consolidating system of for-profit academic publishers. These corporations have been able to reap extreme profits precisely at a time when cuts, precarity, and student debt are being imposed on higher education systems around the world.[94]

Swartz's intervention was not an isolated act of disobedience. It was part of a larger response from readers, scholars, and activists to how common knowledge got locked away. For instance, the Rameshwari Photocopy Services made history when it successfully defended itself in an Indian court against a copyright infringement case brought by a consortium of Oxford University Press, Cambridge University Press, and Taylor & Francis Group. The consortium alleged the service had manufactured unauthorized course packs for professors at the Delhi School of Economics.[95] A banner made by student activists protesting in support of Rameshwari summarized the power asymmetry at play by daring the corporate plaintiffs: "We have the photocopies. Sue us instead along with the Indian Education System! Sue everybody who cannot afford to buy your books."

Protests like this continue at a time when copyright, rather than evolving for the benefit of readers and authors, has entrenched itself further in the name of corporate profits. The shift from print to digital networks vastly increased access to artistic and scientific works, but public libraries, once central in providing access to written culture and knowledge in the print era, were restricted from providing similar access to digital content. Until the mid-2010s, copyright holders blocked libraries from lending digital works, allowing platforms like Google, Amazon, and Elsevier to control digital distribution.[96] The global publishing industry is dominated by ten multinational publishers, with academic publishing alone worth US$20 billion and concentrated among five companies with profit margins as high as 40 percent.[97] These journals, up to 75 percent funded by public or non-profit institutions, rely on researchers who write, review, and edit for these publishers on time paid by the same institutions.[98] Despite public funding, these journals use copyright to lock away knowledge, charging high subscription or open-access processing fees that even well-funded universities struggle to afford.

... and how we take it back

In response, readers, scholars, and activists across the world have taken to digitizing and sharing texts themselves, creating their own piratical systems of access. The sharing of texts is being organized through email lists, Facebook groups ("Ask for PDFs people with institutional Access"), Twitter hashtags ("#ICanHazPDF"), or Telegram and WhatsApp groups; but its principal infrastructure are shadow libraries.[99] These include (at the time of writing) Library Genesis, Science Hub, Anna's Archive, and in a more conceptual key, Aaaaarg. fail, Ubuweb, Monoskop, and our own project, Memory of the World.

Arguably, the most transformative of shadow libraries has been Science Hub, which provides public access to tens of millions of scientific articles that are usually only legally available to academic institutions and individuals who can pay extortionate fees. Science Hub was created in 2011 by Alexandra Elbakyan, then a computer science student in Kazakhstan. A couple of years earlier, Elbakyan developed a script to circumvent paywalls to access articles her school could not afford. After fellow students repeatedly asked her to find articles on their behalf, she set up a website that functions as a search engine and a repository to retrieve paywalled articles. Seven years later, Science Hub provides access to over 60 million, or around 85 percent of all articles behind paywalls, largely fulfilling requests from low- and middle-income countries.[100]

Elbakyan holds the view that science is grounded in the "common ownership of knowledge (i.e. communism) and that copyright should be abolished."[101] She has upheld the principle that the right of the public to access scientific knowledge trumps private property, acting in the Swartzian tradition of civil disobedience to articulate her position.

Shadow libraries are under a constant threat of takedown, and disobedient librarians are under constant risk of prosecution. A lawsuit against Elbakyan by Elsevier was launched in 2015, with penalties potentially running into tens of millions of dollars. Science Hub has had a number of its domains revoked over recent years, but Elbakyan has nonetheless managed to keep its trove of liberated articles accessible. Yet the future of Science Hub, as of this writing, remains uncertain.

Although the prominence of Swartz and Elbakyan might suggest that shadow librarianship is a rare act of defiance, in fact, digitizing, sharing, and maintaining infrastructures are vernacular practices of many, reproducing communities of reading, writing, and thinking across the globe. As a number of us shadow librarians wrote in 2015, in an open letter in solidarity with Science Hub and Library Genesis, these are all practices of custodianship, of curating, of caring for our knowledge commons in defiance of the intellectual property regime.[102] Millions of anonymous people share texts illegally every day, performing quotidian acts of property abolition. They are custodians, too, not only of common knowledge but of a pirate tradition.

Study as disobedient sociality

Just as learning is a fundamental dimension of radical care, disobedience is the lifeblood of radical learning. This principle pulses through Paulo Freire's *Pedagogy of the Oppressed* and bell hooks's *Teaching to Trangress*. It echoes in the actions of Francisco Ferrer, the Spanish anarchist behind the Modern School movement, who saw rebellion as a "natural and rational" force of equality.[103] It is reflected in the philosophy of Loris Malaguzzi, founder of the Reggio Emilia model of early childhood education, who urged educators to assess children not by their compliance, but by their capacity to resist and rebel against conformity.[104]

The practices of radical pedagogy at the heart of disobedient care are about cultivating skills that can help us break molds that society has cast us in and explore what may lie beyond. Fred Moten and Stefano Harney capture this beautifully in their work, where they suggest that our relationship to the university (and other institutions) today must be a "criminal" one. They argue that while the university may offer refuge, it also stifles true individual and collective growth and liberation, forcing us to "sneak in and steal what we can."[105] Their concept of "black study" thus extends beyond accessibility or content alone, to encompass a profound commitment to each other, to the collective, embodied process of learning in defiance of the gatekeepers of knowledge.

In the decade since they published *The Undercommons*, "academic freedom" has nosedived: in 22 countries, including major countries like India, the USA, and China, it has significantly declined, impacting more than half the world's population.[106] Teachers, who should be the custodians of free inquiry, are now facing criminalization for simply discussing critical issues like gender, evolution, or slavery and its afterlives. Meanwhile, managerial policies increasingly dictate not only what teachers teach but also how they shape activities in the classroom, forcing them to do more with less. It's a stark reminder of the escalating crackdown on emancipatory and critical pedagogies, and the importance of continuing to fight for spaces where studying together can be experienced.

Imperial and authoritarian power have historically policed content and access to knowledges, often operating under the paternalistic rhetoric of care for the state, the social order, or moral values. The examples of this specific regime of criminalization targeting educational initiatives are countless, as are indeed the forms of resistance to it. These include the Freedom Schools set up by the Civil Rights Movement in the 1960s in the South of the USA to organize African Americans, the Amílcar Cabral Schools established by the African Party for the Independence of Guinea and Cape Verde (PAIGC) during the liberation struggle of the 1960s and 1970s, the Flying University in mid-1860s Poland, and the study circles for women in post-revolution Iran.

Forms of underground and insurgent education are abundant in our time and are one of the most practiced forms of gathering across resistance movements. A contemporary example of a pirate pedagogy set up to reach excluded groups (here again, women) can be found in Afghanistan, where in the wake of the Taliban's return to power in 2021 after nearly two decades of imperial occupation, access to formal education for girls above 12 has been heavily restricted. Despite the oppressive environment, an underground education movement, referred to as the "schools that don't exist," emerged.[107] Supported by local communities, these networks of clandestine schools offer a range of courses, from English and math to computer skills, and serve over 3,000 students, most often young women. Advanced students often become teachers, creating a ripple effect of knowledge dissemination. These covert educational hubs also feature discrete spaces, such as DIY gyms, defying the physical exercise bans for women. These secret schools symbolize an inspiring Afghan feminist resilience, challenging global narratives that portray these women merely as victims.

Pirate pedagogies, care ecologies

In its current form, education is often a tool for maintaining the status quo, teaching obedience and replicating existing social hierarchies. It cares more for systems than students or communities. But radical pedagogy settings can flip this script, transforming learning into a collective effort grounded in mutual aid and resistance. From this perspective, nurseries and kindergartens, far from being neutral spaces, are spaces where the foundations of social control or rebellion are laid. These are the pedagogical settings where not only children, but their parents and caregivers too, can be subtly indoctrinated into classism, ableism, sexism, racism, and speciesism, and where the family—especially mothers—are re-conscripted as the main providers of intergenerational care labor.

Struggles over early childhood spaces exist at the crossroads of socialization, care, and education. This was made strikingly clear in 2011, when activists occupied a NatWest bank branch in London and transformed it into a temporary childcare center. Their action was one of over 40 temporary occupations of banks across Britain, coordinated by UK Uncut, which re-purposed branches to function as laundries, libraries, homeless shelters, walk-in clinics, and more, in protest against the massive bonuses granted to banks' executives while public services were being drastically defunded. By turning a space of finance into a space of care, protesters reminded us that the revolution might begin in the most unexpected places, and in the shared work of raising a new generation. Sadly, even in radical and leftist scenes, an underestimation of the political significance of intergenerational care, which is often dismissed as "women's work," is still widespread.

Yet, kindergartens are interesting sites to consider from a pirate care perspective. Early childhood education is an area heavily regulated by the state and coveted by religious organizations as sites of recruitment. An increasingly expanding market profits from the fears and hopes of parents, who are encouraged to see their offspring as investments and tasked with sacrificing now to enroll them in highly-ranked educational institutions to enhance their "human capital" and future employability. This tendency, of course, only reinforces hierarchies of racialized and class exclusion while making these appear to be the fault of families and caregivers. In austere times, an increasing number of children are excluded even from publicly funded kindergartens, as public schooling buckles under the weight of cuts. These cuts in public education spending result in overworked teachers, decrepit infrastructure, and dwindling services that cater to children's diverse needs.

This situation has prompted renewed attention to commoning strategies for looking after the youngest, especially from the ranks of those with dependents who fall off the capitalist matrix of care in one or more of three ways: by failing to meet the bureaucratic requirements for accessing public kindergartens, perhaps because they are denied legal status and do not score high enough for a scarce public placement; by failing to earn enough to pay for private childcare; or by living lives outside the normative family structure, for example, in queer families or collectives.

Among the responses we found the recent example of Soprasotto, a self-organized kindergarten opened in Milan in 2013, inspired by the earlier self-managed kindergarten of Porta Ticinese, an initiative born from the radical feminist movements of the 1970s. The Soprasotto collective is made up of educators, parents, and kids. They published an online manual titled "How to Build a Pirate Kindergarten in Your Neighbourhood" aimed at helping others develop their own methods of participatory governance and reflexive practice, but also crucially providing tips on navigating the complex and expensive bureaucratic procedures that can create legal troubles for such communal childcare practices.[108]

In Barcelona, the similar phenomenon of *grupos de crianza compartida* (groups of shared parenting) has gained traction in recent years, setting up informal networks for the commoning of childcare. The practice meets urgent needs of precarious and migrant parents who are cut off from public services yet cannot afford private kindergartens. Despite their critical role, these initiatives found themselves caught in a double bind: when applying for funding, they have been rejected as not diverse enough (in terms of class and background) or not feminist enough (they are largely run by mothers) to meet the relevant criteria.[109] This bureaucratic gatekeeping highlights the contradictory expectations placed upon such initiatives, where their radical potential is often dismissed.

A particularly telling example of the complexities and contradictions inherent in these kinds of initiatives is Koko Lepo, an autonomous kindergarten active in Belgrade from 2013 to 2016. It emerged from the collaboration between anarchist activists of the InexFilm squat in the Karaburma neighborhood and the Roma families in the informal settlement Deponija mahala. This initiative sought to bridge the deep-seated social, racial, and class divides between these two constituencies and faced significant challenges. Within the InexFilm collective, some members were more focused on cultural activities and did not recognize the value of a children's program. Externally, Koko Lepo was criticized as providing a "service" to Roma people, which risked reproducing paternalistic dynamics. Despite these setbacks, Koko Lepo's refusal to seek official status as an NGO was a crucial element of fostering accountability in the context of extreme antiziganist (anti-Romani) sentiments.

Elsewhere, access to childcare has been reimagined as a key ingredient of militant protests, as in the 2020 Yard Movement in Minsk, Belarus. An anonymous member of the Museum of Stones Collective put it this way:

> People would leave their children to one of the apartments and they would assign turns so that people would look after the children one after another, so in that way they would free up time for people to do either activist work or to do their normal job, or to take time and go help their family members . . .[110]

The Yard Movement gained momentum during the anti-government protests in Belarus in 2020, establishing an impressive pirate care infrastructure in response to the parallel threats of political repression and the COVID-19 pandemic. This movement takes its name after Minsk's residential courtyards. After the government disabled the internet on the first night of political unrest on August 9, 2020, many people gathered outside to stay informed. This marked the beginning of a new way of connecting neighbors. As the government preemptively blocked central squares and brutally suppressed and criminalized dissidents, the movement shifted to decentralized gatherings in residential yards.

The events in the yards were not always overtly political but addressed the needs of the collective "fragile body." They included concerts, games, readings, yard tea parties, and childcare, showing how the circuits of the "yard economy" were created "not only to make pressure, but also to create joy."[111] Political undertones were ever present, driven by the community's urge to resist repression and stay connected. With the government controlling all media and frequent internet shutdowns, printed newspapers and posters, often placed in mailboxes, were crucial for spreading information. Even before the protests, residents organized around essential needs. The tap water contamination in a Minsk district on 24 June 2020, and the government's silence for three days, first prompted grassroots initiatives for water distribution. Supported by an online map showing availability, this effort laid the groundwork for the later yard movement, demonstrating the power of local self-organization.

Partisan expertise

In messy territories of confrontation, where persecuted populations develop forms of mass intellectuality, we frequently see the emergence of what we will call "partisan expertise." A salient feature of the partisan knowledges is their ability to bridge local struggles with broader insurgencies against the mutating forms of sovereignty of Empire. A recent example is the NO TAV movement in Northern Italy, where activists, deeply tied to their landscape, have conducted their own geological studies to contest the government's plans for an ecologically and socially destructive high-speed rail link between France and Italy.[112] Or we might consider the protagonism of ACT UP in the US during the peak of the AIDS epidemic, where activists became deeply knowledgeable about the drug approval processes their lives depended on, challenging both the pharmaceutical industry and the government's failures.[113] In cases such as these, activists embrace their role as generators of a unique kind of knowledge, one that emerges from the terrain, the body, and the urgent need to resist. Their "partisan expertise" is born from an intimate connection and commitment to study their condition and its place in the world. This common knowledge is both a tool of survival and a means of reimagining what is possible.

Earlier in this book, we emphasized a politics of care that requires a commitment not only to caring for carers but also for their tools—whether books, online platforms, toys, or other resources. However, when discussing partisan expertise, we must be careful not to reduce knowledge to its cognitive aspects alone. What makes this expertise truly partisan is its deep connection to collective bodies and specific places, and the vital role of affect in the politics of care and its pedagogy. Every form of education carries a hidden curriculum, shaping behaviors and relationships as much as it trains skills. The sociality of partisan expertise sustains different ways of belonging and differentiating. Partisan expertise yanks the rug out from under the feet of those who tout neutral, professionalized, and supposedly "only" technical interventions.

5

Organizing Mutiny to Mutualize Care

The Golden Age of pirates in the eighteenth century saw these "villains of all nations" thrive in a context of inter-imperialist rivalry. But while kingdoms of Europe vied for supremacy, they shared a common commitment to the exploitation of the world and its people, justified by religious dogma that celebrated the sovereignty and the patriarchal family as God's intended social forms. In this context, pirate crews, who composed themselves from mutinied sailors, runaway servants, enslaved people who liberated themselves and other vagabonds, challenged the imperial order not only through the dangers they posed to merchants on high seas but also in the way they reinvented family and kinship in defiance of the patriarchal, colonial, and white supremacist norms of the day.

Female pirates like Anne Bonny and Mary Read evaded execution by "pleading their bellies," a strategic claim of pregnancy that stayed their execution, a survival tactic that was a mocking commentary on the state's grip on life and death. Similarly, anthropologist David Graeber reveals a fascinating legacy of unconventional alliances forged between multiracial pirates and Malagasy women who, excluded from power by patriarchal structures of their tribes, strategically leveraged their relationships with these desperate (but often well-armed) interlopers to disrupt local patriarchal regimes.[114] They played a pivotal role in channeling pirate wealth into the local economy, while simultaneously transmitting values of equality and democracy from pirate ships into Malagasy society. In so doing, they crafted an interracial, intercultural form of self-governance that challenged the racialized and gendered hierarchies of both imperial and traditional rule.

Another fascinating aspect of pirate sociality was the practice of "matelotage," a form of queer intimacy that blurred lines between camaraderie, romantic desire, and strategic alliance. These civil partnerships involved pirates forming close bonds, sharing possessions, and providing for each other as spouses. These relationships offered a radical alternative to European norms, allowing pirates to create their own structures of queer and intergenerational care.

Today, reactionary nostalgia for "traditional" family structures mystifies care work as a gendered act of love. This comes at exactly the same time as many families increasingly rely on the cheapened labor of maids, cleaners, and personal carers (mostly migrant women) to cover for the retreat of the welfare state and the increased costs of living, which requires more breadwinners.

In addressing the possibilities of pirate care in the domestic terrain, we follow the lead of Indigenous and queer struggles, who use the terms of kinship to politicize intimate relations. What is at stake in kinning practices is the forging of reliable expectations of care that contain promises of mutuality not based on what is already in common, but on commitment. Kinning describes the cultivation of forms of care that augment the freedom of others (to recall Graeber's definition of care), others who are not-quite-like-us, yet whose freedom and well-being determine ours. What is more, in kinship bonds there is an invocation of reciprocity that is not symmetrical and that cannot be inscribed in an economy of exchange. It defies the regime of self-interested exchanges that defines Empire's state–market–family matrix of care.

Within that matrix, current care institutions are centered on the artificial but beguiling institutions of the cisheteronormative family and the private household. Even public institutions defer to family for consent, custody, or financial responsibility, often ignoring needs of those estranged from family or reliant on non-normative bonds for support. Within private households, care is structured by patriarchal norms: tasks of cleaning, cooking, rearing kids, or looking after the elderly are performed predominantly by women, a division of labor essential for capitalist accumulation, as it undervalues and invisibilizes the care labor that sustains daily life and the economy.[115]

Against this backdrop, there is some unique traction at stake in the queer activation of "political kinship." As Lisa Beard described, instead of "turning toward the state," the invocation of kinship "creates conditions for and forges practices of turning toward each other."[116] This is indeed a core possibility of pirate care: the skillful creation of forms of entrustment that can sustain, through continued everyday gestures, communities of practice and registers of political belonging that are not striving to be assimilated or guaranteed or superseded by the state.

Queering as in kinning

Care is structured around the patriarchal cisheteronormative family and, in turn, cisheteronormativity is often enforced through the denial of care, often with tragic consequences. According to US data, four in five transgender people have seriously considered, and two in five have attempted, suicide.[117] Conversion therapy, a banned method of attempting to change a person's gender identity to cisgender, is still allowed in most countries.

In the late 1960s and early 1970s, New York trans activists Sylvia Rivera and Marsha P. Johnson established the STAR House. It was part of a groundbreaking moment in which the trans community asserted itself as a force with radical insights on how society might better organize care beyond mere survival.[118] The story of the Street Transvestite Action Revolutionaries House (STAR House) began in a trailer truck in the East Village, serving as both a shelter and a social space for trans and unhoused LGBTIQ+ youth. This initial setup laid the groundwork for what would become a more permanent home at 213 East Second Street, a dilapidated building in a "bad neighborhood" with no basic amenities. Despite these challenging beginnings, Rivera and Johnson (both in their 20s) and their comrades transformed this space into a livable refuge. They did so through many forms of resourceful ingenuity, aiming to ensure safety and care for their chosen family. They assumed the roles of mothers as a key technique of entrustment between different generations of queer youth. Rivera is reported to have corrected a newcomer who addressed her by her first name: "Oh no, honey," Sylvia admonished, "you don't call me Sylvia no more. I'm your mother. You call me Ma."[119] The importance of this performative hack cannot be underestimated in a context where LGBTIQ+ individuals were denied the guidance and care of elders in their lives. Rivera and Johnson created a "safe space" in the unforgiving heart of a society that sought to erase them. Unlike communes in the countryside, STAR operated in direst urban conditions, mirroring the legacy of activist mothers in African American communities, who have long provided mutual aid under extreme poverty and repression. As bell hooks highlighted, "homeplace" has always been a site of resistance for Black people in the US.[120] "Othermothering" in Black communities extended care beyond biological boundaries to nurture the collective.[121]

At its core, then, the STAR House was an embodiment of radical affective and material care, where the idea of mothering is detached from its arbitrary association with biology and gender. While Rivera and Johnson, as Mothers, engaged in sex work, they were adamant about ensuring that the youth in their care were not compelled by circumstance, as many trans people are, to pursue this line of work. "We didn't want the kids out in the streets hustling," Rivera confided to writer Leslie Feinberg. To keep the cupboards stocked, the House's children rather resorted to shoplifting, wryly re-formulated as "Fingers for Jesus," a euphemism inspired by Rivera's friend, Reverend Pat Bumgardner.

Sousveillance against police

Indigenous theorists, including Leanne Simpson and Kim Tallbear, remind us how non-normative kinship ties provide a vital organizing framework in struggles for anticolonial sovereignty and ecological care. Traditional and innovative Indigenous practices of nonmonogamy, gender fluidity, and community child-rearing are systematically undermined by colonial forces, and indeed their legal and moral prohibition has long been a key weapon in the colonial arsenal. Indigenous kinning, like Black cultural practices of polymaternalism, offer a generative genealogy for a radical politics of care.

Wiindo Debwe Mosewin Patrol, translating to "Walking in Truth," represents a profound reimagining of community safety, through kinship and collective care initiated by Indigenous activists in Thunder Bay, Ontario, a city with among the highest per capita Indigenous population in Canada. Here, Indigenous people face a daily onslaught of dangers: human trafficking, police brutality, and racially motivated violence, all of which compound systemic racism that manifests in poverty, poor health, and criminalization.[122] The city is infamous for "starlight tours," where police officers abandon Indigenous people on the outskirts, often after stripping them of life saving clothing. This is deadly in a place where temperatures regularly dip below −30C.

In response, Wiindo Debwe Mosewin Patrol was born. Comprised of about 40 volunteers, the Patrol makes circuits of the streets, waterways, bridges, and woods of Thunder Bay, searching for those in distress. In a context where two independent investigations found the police to be systemically racist and where most Indigenous people have experienced or heard firsthand accounts of police violence, these volunteers operate outside of the purview of colonial institutions. They practice what Ivory Tuesday, one of the groups' spokespeople, has termed a practice of "sousveillance," inspired by Black feminist scholar Simone Brown's description of how oppressed groups reverse power dynamics by monitoring actions of those in positions of authority.[123]

Volunteers patrol dangerous areas, offering rides to those who might otherwise be left vulnerable to attack by the police or racists. They also confront the physical symbols of hate, such as by painting over racist graffiti. They are often met with slurs or even physical intimidation by groups of white men, encouraged by their supporters in positions of authority. These acts of resistance are deeply intertwined with Anishinaabe cultural practices: before painting over hate-filled messages, the patrollers smudge, burning ceremonial herbs to cleanse the space and reclaim it as a site of Indigenous presence.

Central to Wiindo Debwe Mosewin's philosophy is the concept of "two-eyed seeing," which involves drawing on both Indigenous traditions and settler ways of knowing and being. This approach allows them to practice what they call "contextual fluidity," adapting to the needs of the moment while remaining rooted in their cultural traditions. The Moccasin Telegram, an Indigenous oral tradition that has evolved into a modern network of digital communication, is another key element of this practice. Through this grassroots method, the Wiindo Debwe Mosewin collective anonymously shares stories, alerting the community to dangers, and documenting instances of racist violence that are ignored by the media.

Kinship organizing in uncharted waters

M. E. O'Brien argues that, since the onset of imperial industrial capitalism, the nuclear family has served as a machine for producing and reproducing the working class.[124] Initially, this was achieved by breaking up pre-existing kin relationships and imposing the home-owning male breadwinner family as the model to aspire to. After WWII, the working class fought to achieve this model, only to see it erode in the 1970s as wages declined, forcing housewives into the labor market to help make ends meet. The material economy's dependence on the nuclear family had its moral economic counterpart: coercing people into strict gender roles, enlisting women as primary care workers, policing Black families to conform to white norms, and criminalizing Indigenous kinship.[125] Although the erosion of the nuclear family model has, to a certain extent, increased toleration for diverse family forms (including single-parent, queer, and intergenerational families), the flourishing of the private household remains the material basis of capitalist reproduction, and white, male, property-owning individualism continues to dominate as the ideological standard. In this context, a number of pirate care techniques address the harm of existing care structures, opening up new possibilities of healing and autonomy.

An example of this is "Stand-in Pride," an initiative providing temporary surrogate family members for significant life events, such as weddings or graduations. This initiative was started by Daniel Blevins, who first gained attention in January 2021 with a TikTok video offering to be a "stand-in dad" for LGBTIQ+ couples whose biological parents were unsupportive or absent at their weddings. This idea rapidly evolved, leading to the creation of a Facebook group that has grown to over 36,000 members across more than 70 countries. In an era of uprootedness and alienation, it aims to support LGBTIQ+ people with physical presence and emotional backing of others at important life events, helping build "chosen family" relationships.

Likewise, The Hologram, a platform for grassroots care, originally devised in 2017 by Cassie Thornton as an art project but now run collectively, uses both online and in-person meetings to refuse the capitalist matrix of care.[126] This deceptively simple protocol, where three people meet with and provide care for a fourth, was inspired by a practice generated by one of the more radical Greek Solidarity Clinics discussed in the first chapter. In 2011, a clinic in Thessaloniki started an experiment where each new patient met simultaneously with a doctor, a psychotherapist, and a social worker or community activist. These three figures would conduct a shared interview with the "incomer" (they refused the conventional medical terms like "patient") to gather a more holistic "three-dimensional" record of the conditions impacting their well-being (hence, the name hologram), grasping not only physical, but also psychosocial and political determinants of their health.

The Hologram practice begins with a person (a hologram) inviting three people (a triangle), who could be friends or acquaintances but also strangers, to commit to supporting her by regularly meeting up to discuss her physical, psychic, and social health. Thornton explains that her motivation stemmed from observing conditions she and her friends experienced, where "everyone is a little sick" under capitalism. This belief was shared by another contributor to the Pirate Care Syllabus, Power Makes us Sick (PMS), a collective dedicated to autonomous medicine and herbalism.[127] While PMS primarily organizes practices within anarchist movements, offering medical care in situations of police clashes or supporting longer processes of healing activist burnouts, the emphasis of the Hologram is to provide a mutual support system to "dehabituate" us from the capitalist belief that care is scarce and that to ask to be cared for is somewhat shameful. To bootstrap that process, Thornton and Lita Wallis have developed training courses to initiate the practice, and these teaching materials can be found in the Pirate Care Syllabus.

In a different context, but with a shared emphasis on repoliticizing care, efforts in Abya Yala focus on reclaiming intimate bonds through feminist self-defense. The recent Ni Una Menos uprisings mobilized millions in Chile, Argentina, Mexico, and other South American countries to resist the violent patriarchy that results in over 4,000 femicides each year.[128] As Colectivo ADA (Acción Directa Autogestiva) clarified in a 2017 communiqué,

> feminist self-defense consists not only of practicing a martial art, but also of creating safe spaces, collective self-care and affective networks, and of thinking about violence in all its forms and developing counter-strategies.[129]

In the same context, since the spring of 2015, the Laboratory of Interconnectivities and Hummingbird Command have converged in the Hackfeminist Self-Defense project in Oaxaca, Mexico. Through their workshops, gatherings, and training sessions, they have, they report, "developed a strategic methodology of hybridizing martial arts techniques, feminist self-defense, and digital collective care." What is distinctive in this cyberfeminist approach, which extends tactical separatist and consciousness-raising repertoires, is the way facilitators refuse to uphold the distinction "between online and offline" spaces, understanding that both dimensions impact the well-being of women. In this sense, the body is seen as "our first technology" and communal sessions as "an affective-generative algorithm."[130] This underscores a key theme of this book: since we live in a post-digital world where online violence supercharges physical violence, we do not gain much in treating these realms as separate. As they counter violence equally in virtual and physical spaces, as extensions of each other, Hackfeminist Self-Defense activists place mutual care at the center of a political rethinking of our relation with technologies.

Care-fully hacking familial laws

One distinct approach to pirate care and kinning hacks the laws that are meant to define and confine family. A significant yet under-researched example of this tactic is the practice of same-sex adult adoption: the legal adoption of an adult partner aimed at securing legal benefits such as inheritance rights, tax advantages, and hospital visitation privileges. For many years, and more visibly since the 1970s and 1980s, adopting an adult partner to establish them as a legal heir was strategically employed out of necessity in a legal landscape that offered few alternatives to same-sex couples. Notable examples include Marina Cicogna, an Italian film producer who legally adopted her younger partner, Benedetta, out of á lack of other options and, in the US, the case of the civil rights organizer Bayard Rustin, coordinator of logistics for the Martin Luther

King Jr.'s March on Washington, who adopted his partner Walter Naegle in 1982.

However, hacking this legal tool forces participants to face a number of complex legal and moral dilemmas: one cannot divorce one's heir if the relationship ends, and an adoptee must sever their legal relationship with their previous parents. As laws change to permit same-sex unions, those who once relied on adult adoption now find themselves in legal limbo, often at the mercy of individual judges.

The state's institution of marriage has also been hacked by activists challenging anti-immigration policies. An illustration is the Protection Marriage project, initiated by German artist and activist Silke Wagner. The project primarily takes the form of a multi-lingual website offering detailed instructions to successfully arrange what the European Union calls "fictitious marriages": those intended to defy immigration regulations. In this case, these marriages are intended to allow those fleeing persecution or danger to stay legally in countries that afford greater safety or opportunity. Wagner leveraged the freedom often afforded to artistic expression to provide practical information and implicitly to encourage the practice of protection marriage. We can describe this as a kind of pirate art, building on the proud tradition of manipulating appearances, loopholes, and the grey areas of the law to retake space for renegade solidarities.

The Protection Marriage project unfolds an oblique critique of the institution of marriage and its entanglement with the state. The guide underscores the precariousness of those in need of such marriages and questions the state's intrusions into the sphere of intimate relations. It also relates a number of interviews with individuals involved in such marriages. In one such interview, Fatima and Bernd discuss the labor that these unions entail in order to negotiate bureaucratic whirlpools and emotional complexities. Bernd explains his motivations:

> I have been involved with anti-racism for years and have seen again and again how people can be pushed around and deported . . . Protection Marriage was, to this extent, always a necessary and justified option for me. I also see it as a possibility and privilege to use my German passport in a meaningful way.

Fatima articulates the impact of the carceral migration system: "During this time the situation affected me psychologically . . . But with marriage it was immediately different."

Protection Marriage invites its audiences to reflect on the concrete ways of practicing solidarity, redistribution, and affective care between those who act from "low-intensity, low-risk and low-stakes struggles" and those whose conditions are high-intensity, high-risk, and high-stakes.[131] Some of these concrete ways emerge in struggles, such as when white protesters deliberately put themselves in the way of cops at demonstrations for Black lives, or in the role of anti-Zionist Jews in pro-Palestinian struggles. Others operate across greater distances/differences, like the Phone

Credit for Refugees, which crowdsources funds to pay for cell phone bills and internet data for undocumented migrants on the move.

Despite their diversity, we believe these practices all create opportunities for people to collaborate in making those most vulnerable to police, state, and market violence safer in their resistance. They do so without relying upon professionalized NGOs, state agencies, or religious intermediaries. These forms of pirate care politicize our power imbalances and privilege, in defiance of laws and norms that uphold the patriarchal family's monopoly on care.

A call to mutiny

In this chapter, we have traced the contours of radical kinship through both the anarchic praxis of eighteenth-century pirates, the radical heydays of trans liberation in the 1960s, and the audacious re-imaginings of care by present-day Indigenous and queer communities. While not all of these examples strictly break the law, they all fiercely transgress moral norms that routinely humiliate and hurt people who reject the patriarchal family as the primary unit of care.

That patriarchal family is presented in state, market, and religious propaganda as a lonely ship in a stormy world, the only reliable source of real security on the high seas of an austere and uncaring society. The reality is that this ship is not just sinking; it was never seaworthy to begin with. It was constructed within and in the service of a capitalist economy that values individuals not as agents of their own narratives but as units of labor—waged or domestic(ated). The family is not just failing, it is already self-abolishing, leaving behind a trail of broken expectations, reactionary nostalgia, and toxic modes of caring and uncaring.

This is why we wish to end this chapter with a call to mutiny. Marriage dissolution rates, the widespread "heteropessimistic" despair of people of all genders within heteronormative confines, the disillusionment with romantic ideals, and the chronic intergenerational tensions found within conventional family setups all speak to a profound dissonance between lived realities and imposed norms. But these realities alone don't necessarily threaten the cruel optimism of the family (with a heartfelt nod to Lauren Berlant). In an austere, uncaring world, the promise of the family, with its easily consumed norms and relations, is addictive. When we reflect on the possibilities of organizing our intimate and domestic lives through the prism of pirate care, we come to realize that more than mere allies, we need to become accomplices to one another.

However, in our enthusiasm to celebrate forms of defiance against the patriarchal family, we must guard against approaches that harm or blame mothers (regardless of their gender). We must also be wary of the ways in which the language of kinship can be used coercively. Even within militant circles, the vocabulary of family and kinship have often been employed to maintain unequal power dynamics as well as exploitative roles and gendered expectations within collectives. A sharp reminder of the perils of invoking familial relations also comes to us via the history of the feminist movement, where white middle-class feminist mobilizations of notions of sisterhood or trade unionist notions of brotherhood served to hide and marginalize anti-racist struggles. As Sophie Lewis provocatively put it, the family is indeed a seductive "technology of privatization" not only of wealth, but crucially, of care.

As we explore the role of criminalized kinning practices in today's social movements, we must recognize that their political relevance lies in their function within broader revolutionary struggles. Practicing new forms of kinship must be rooted in a relentless commitment to structural changes that can also impact those with whom we do not share an affinity. In other words, they must transform society and its material bases, not just immediate social relations; and these goals must be inter-twined. These kinship practices cannot serve us as cozy substitutes for broader struggles. They can and should be micropolitical manifestations where the libidinal drives for a liberated future are rehearsed, nurtured, and made militant.

In this spirit, the call for mutiny in this chapter is a reminder that we need to cultivate tech-niques for capturing the kin-ship and re-orienting it toward the uncharted waters of a better future for all. As we confront the leviathan of Empire's matrix of care, we recognize that these structures no longer serve us, if indeed they ever did. They anchor us to bigoted fantasies of middle-class domestic bliss and consumerist escapism that will not fulfill us, and that threaten the planet's ecological capacities.

The task ahead is monumental, but it is also exhilarating, and full of care.

Conclusion
Swearing an Oath

In this book we have offered dozens of examples of contemporary and historical pirate care practices in fields as diverse as housing, farming, healthcare, childcare, transcare, migration, and infrastructure. In a world where acts of solidarity are increasingly criminalized and delegitimated, it is crucial for militants to understand the logic underpinning Empire's matrix of care and the way it contributes to our miseries. The acts we analyzed are not undertaken out of sympathy or charity, but as creative and insurrectionary acts of self-organized support, repair, healing, and militant autonomy. They advance from a fundamental belief that the system of profit-driven and state-sanctioned death must be opposed. By defying both the seductive and the repressive aspects of the state, the market, and the family, pirate care is a prefigurative mode of struggle, carving out a future that refuses privatized care and insists on a commonist horizon based on the radical redistribution of nurture.

When considered in isolation, individual pirate care initiatives may not seem to offer a comprehensive political "solution." They respond to urgent, palpable needs right in front of them. Yet, what we hope to have demonstrated is that through the very practice of formulating, reformulating, and continuously calibrating their responses, a political horizon is emerging. Pirate care is already happening in a myriad of places, as people provide care to one another out of necessity in defiance of the dominant order. However, these scattered initiatives rarely recognize themselves as part of an incipient revolutionary challenge to that order, helping us see beyond the scarcity, legalism, and property relations at the heart of Empire.

These acts of immediate pirate care might be among the most effective challenges to capitalism today. Autonomously organized care initiatives with the ambition to federate present a terrifying prospect to capital accumulation because they give us the capacity to reproduce life and resistance under expanding conditions of freedom. They allow us to remove ourselves from a reliance on the state, the market, or the family. Like the pirates of old, these are acts of renegade carers reclaiming their capacity to make worlds. That's why they are criminalized: the common wealth that they produce nourishes and propagates other forms of struggle. As they multiply, diversify, and connect, their collective power grows to more than the sum of its parts. While no one initiative or struggle is dominant, they complement one another to make each one stronger. They thus allow for a revolutionary reclamation of society and its institutions.

By highlighting care's associations with acts of piracy and disobedience, we aim to reclaim care as a force for transformative change, transcending mere symbolic gestures and fostering radical political engagement rooted in the material realities of the fraught world we inhabit. Pirate care practices offer a pragmatic mode of conduct that can help movements sidestep moralisms that are organized around the fantasy of purity. While the term solidarity is often used to describe many experiences of aiding others, it is important to understand that this term carries a specific political meaning, describing a conscious decision to partake in the vulnerability that is imposed on someone else. This condition of shared vulnerability, rooted in the recognition of our fragile bodies, and the abolition of systemic injustices, is the starting point for a pirate politics of solidarity.

This understanding of solidarity demonstrates why pirate care practices should not be confused with humanitarianism. As Pia Klemp, a Sea-Watch boat captain, aptly warned,

I'm not a humanitarian. I am not there to "aid." I stand in with you in solidarity. We do not need medals. We do not need authorities deciding about who is a "hero" and who is "illegal." In fact, they are in no position to make this call because we are all equal.[132]

We must acknowledge that right-wing movements also provide care. In the 1920s, Nazi soup kitchens for wounded soldiers doubled as recruitment centers. Today, conservative and far-right institutions embed themselves within communities by offering care, stitching themselves into the social fabric. This underscores the importance of the radical discourse presented in this book, offering carers a more profoundly political narrative to explain their actions in contrast to those forms of care that exclude entire groups of people deemed undeserving of support.

Punitive neoliberalism makes care scarce and criminalizes solidarity in order to keep the system of value extraction and statist social control ticking. But it undercuts the very conditions that make life possible. Amid this, nostalgic welfare chauvinism emerges as a band-aid solution from the capitalist state, an attempt to plaster over the discontent that simmers beneath the surface of society. Meanwhile, the market dons a cloak of philanthropy, a masquerade of care that merely glosses over deep-seated injustices. Both the state and the market uphold the sanctity of the patri-archal nuclear family and private household as untouchable even while they download onto it (particularly onto women) a burden of care that pushes it to the breaking point. These attempts at remedy, offered as a salve to our systemic afflic-tions, now find us trapped in a trilemma, caught between the logics of state, family, and market (often replicated across the third sector, too). Each path leads us further into crisis. Much of society, unprepared for the ongoing failure of these insti-tutions, is now engulfed in a generational panic that fuels the fires of fascism. It often appears that all that remains is resentment, cynicism, and desperation, the sad passions of neoliberal cap-italism, neocoloniality, and patriarchy. Yet this withered landscape is ripe for a radical reimagin-ing of our approach to care and solidarity, fueled by a militant joy.

Drawing from the pirate care practices in this book, we will conclude by unraveling five threads from which we can weave a new political fabric.

The abolitionist instituting of care

Pirate care is rooted in collective action as people organize to transgress laws, mutualize risk, and challenge power. This involves an abolitionist form of instituting that organizes against the violence and routinized neglect stemming from current laws, the bureaucratic death machine, and digitalized chains of command. Rather than giving up on institutions, pirate care embraces plural, abolitionist processes of deinstitutionalization and parallel prefigurative efforts to invent new institutions based on non-coercive and inclusive principles of democratic decision-making, as summarized in the slogans "nothing about us without us" and "no responsibilities without power." These initiatives reject total institutions of care, those that isolate specific populations, either for special treatment or special punishment.

The commoning of private property

Pirate care initiatives fundamentally challenge private property, reclaiming the resources and tools they need to create systems of commoning and meet collective needs. As Empire restructures itself around intellectual property and land grabs, where the sanctity of private property guarantees corporations indemnity for social and ecological depredations, it is crucial for care activism to not only emphasize labor but also integrate a rejection of private property and its regimes. Private property is the real abstraction that binds together the state, the market, and the family and enables

Empire's matrix of care. We must experiment with transforming private property into a common wealth over the means necessary for fostering a world grounded in mutual interdependence.

The critical usership of technology

Pirate carers reappropriate technologies in innovative ways to expand access to resources, subverting dominant technological systems that tend to accelerate social isolation, deskilling, and environmental destruction. This critical usership transcends the urge to avoid technologies or imagine care as "natural" and pre-technological, acknowledging that in our post-digital condition, technologies shape our world and our cooperation, even if we opt out individually. Therefore, we need a critical horizon for technology and knowledge. This cannot be enclosed by techno-solutionist fantasies that promise liberation from toil, want, and hardship but deliver only corporate power. Focusing on tinkering, collective reskilling, and reappropriation can make technologies work for the creative re-organizing of care labor.

The militant embrace of collective learning

Pirate care involves the development and sharing of partisan expertise: knowledge rooted in lived experience that can expand our common understanding of struggles. Such learning must be offered freely and deliberately to empower others. Education is a form of care, both in the sense of learning together and in the sense of passing on knowledge intergenerationally, from struggle to struggle, from militant to militant. We need deep pedagogies that do not position expertise as the opposite of political engagement. Alongside advocating for access to knowledge, we need to push back against the privatization of education and the compromised terrain of educational institutions, but also by refusing to settle for their current limitations and injustices.

The queering of kinning to create new forms of intergenerational life in common

Pirate care initiatives challenge the patriarchal nuclear family as the dominant model for organizing intimate care by embracing and experimenting with kinning processes based on diversity and mutual support. Practices of queer kinning foreground the ways our passions are put to work under the regime of Empire (love, hate, indifference, hopelessness). By complexifying our attachments and affinities, we can question division of responsibilities into private and public and give each other permission to support intimacies that defy conventional roles between people, and between people and the world. But the nurturing of queer affinities and libidinal investments must also be attached to strategic struggles for broader infrastructures of care and to mass-organizing to demand and create care-full democratic institutions that can support diverse populations at scale. They are crucial to the ways we can reimagine and rebuild a world of care that embraces not only our diversity and interdependence, but also our transversal relations to the other-than-human world.

A federation of carers

Pirate care practices reconfigure the terrain of struggles altogether. They are not just acts of disobedience; they have the capacity to actively undermine the cycle of power reproduction at a structural level. Envisioning a pirate federation as a concluding imaginary for us means harnessing the energy liberated from the shackles of mere survival and channeling it into political possibility. This requires creating spaces where we can redefine our subjectivities and build a collective identity rooted in motley, plebeian, and planetary worldmaking.

One of the central ideas of this book is that mutiny is already a shared reality in the landscape of care—a recognition that if we truly wish to care for this world and its inhabitants, we must disobey the orders that bind us to its shipwreck.

Yet, as scary as mutiny might seem, we wish to end these pages by naming what it enables. The federative principle sustains autonomy and mutual obligation within a web of interconnectedness. It's a concept that amplifies power and accountability against dominant hierarchies of the present-day Empire propped up by global financialized capitalism, technological warlordism, and the geopolitical war of attrition that is destroying social and ecological foundations of survival for most of us. This principle was central to the anarchists and communists of the past century and was a guiding light for the Non-Aligned Movement, which, in the 1960s, envisioned an internationalist, anti-colonial world. Today, we witness its practice in Rojava and Chiapas, and in the efforts to reclaim the internet from state and market enclosure through the "federated web." We join in an aspiration to build a global common out of federated communes and commons.

Federation is already implicit in the pirate care practices we've documented, where collective intelligence and coordinated action are key. It also guided our work on the Pirate Care Syllabus, which wasn't tied to a single issue but aimed to connect militant caregivers with a shared ethos, shared strategies, and a shared story. As we wrote this book, federation became our wager. We believe pirate care will expand as Empire's crises of care and life intensify. We will increasingly rely on self-organized care, though the political stakes remain uncertain, and the threat of fascist care looms large.

This is why we hope federation can serve as our shared horizon, to be realized in concrete movements. Pirate care initiatives are inherently fragile; they may not last long. Collectives dissolve, people move on, and the law may swiftly shut us down. But by committing to complement and support other self-governed initiatives, pirate care practices persist, cropping up in new forms and different contexts as needed. Federation offers a way to move beyond disillusionment, to regroup in ways that match the moment without succumbing to cynicism or burnout. This, we hope, is what our book contributes to.

In the Golden Age of Piracy, at the dawn of the European imperial capitalist world, renegade sailors turned pirate and so joined the motley, plebeian worldmaking project of a "hydrarchy from below."[133] On their ships and in their enclaves, pirates constructed democratic, redistributive, egalitarian, and combative multiracial micro-societies against the world of empires. By becoming care pirates today, at the end of an Empire that threatens to take our world down with it, we are conjuring a new "hydrachy from below." We need a pirate code to summon our crew and a witch's spell book to sustain life against all odds. Thus, in offering our book as a tool for sensing and organizing, we leave it in your hands as both a cypher and an invocation—a pledge we make to each other to liberate care in all its political joy, and a spell to hold each other dear as we set sails to take us into the gathering storm.

Acknowledgments

This book is a testament to the queer, ingenuous, and unruly energies of all those who disobey and nurture radical care. It is a fruit borne from a sprawling, feral constellation of kin, lovers, comrades, and accomplices who have, in their myriad ways, midwifed this collective wisdom into being. We begin by spilling our gratitude for the dazzling array of co-conspirators, story weavers, movement builders, facilitators, and fire-stokers who have added to our understanding of what a pirate care could be and do: Laura Benitez Valero, Emina Bužinkić, Rasmus Fleischer, Maddalena Fragnito, Chris Grodotzki and Morana Miljanović at Sea-Watch, Mary Maggic, Iva Marčetić, Power Makes Us Sick (PMS), Paula Pin (Biotranslab/ Pechblenda), Planka, Zoe Romano, Cassie Thornton, Ivory Tuesday, Ana Vilenica, Women on Waves. Thank you for your quotidian refusal to accept the world as it is and for your audacity in re-producing it otherwise. Our thanks go out to Mijke van der Drift, Taraneh Fazeli, Kirsten Forkert, Janna Graham, Victoria Mponda, Toufic Haddad, Jelka Kretzschmar, Franziska Wallner, Gilbert B. Rodman, Deborah Streahle, Nick Titus, Kim Trogal, Kandis Williams, Kitty Worthing, James Skinner, John Wilbanks, who breathed life into the first Pirate Care conference at the Centre for Postdigital Cultures in Coventry in June 2019. Your ideas, your presence, your commitments shaped our initial conversations and let us know how to keep going. To Cooperation Birmingham, Sezonieri, Janneke Adema, Antonia Hernández, Rebekka Kiesewetter, Tobias Steiner, and all the many more amazing contributors and translators of "Flatten the Curve, Grow the Care": thank you for believing in the power of collective witnessing and learning, even as the pandemic scrambled our compasses.

Our deepest gratitude to the folks within the organizations and institutions who supported us, not out of obligation, but from a shared sense of necessity. To the people at WeMake Milan, the Centre for Postdigital Cultures at Coventry University, Drugo More, with special mention to Davor Mišković, Ivana Katić, Petra Corva, and Dubravko Matanić; to Rijeka European Capital of Culture 2020; to Galerija Nova; to the curatorial collective What, How and for Whom and Andrea Hubin at Kunsthalle Wien. Our thanks also go to the folks at Venice Climate Camp, Aksioma, Disruption Network Lab, Acud macht neu & Collective Practices, Media City Film Festival, CRIC—Festival of Critical Culture, Manual Labours, E.A.R. (Education.Arts. Research), Radio Roža, New Alphabet School, Neural, Soundings, and Kulturpunkt. You shared resources and held space for our messy, beautiful gatherings and set in motion so many of the reflections that weave through this manuscript.

A special recognition goes to our Vagabonds: Amanda Priebe and Max Haiven: thank you for your unrelenting encouragement and for making this struggle your own. To Liz Mason-Deese, and Stevphen Shukaitis, for your sharp, witty, and generous inputs. To David Shulman, Robert Webb, Carrie Giunta, Dave Stanford, Emily Orford, Sophie O'Reirdan, Patrick Hughes, Jonila Krasniqi, and the Pluto Press team for shepherding this book and allowing it to take a form true to our practice.

Finally, a fierce embrace to the countless insurgent souls who took the Pirate Care Syllabus and ran with it, pushing it beyond our initial archipelagos and affinities, and to the many more who continue to fight for an ungovernable, joyous care.

Notes

1. Gomperts, Rebecca. "Women on Waves: Where Next for the Abortion Boat?" *Reproductive Health Matters* 10, no. 19 (May 2002): 180–83.

2. Hardt, Michael, and Antonio Negri. *Empire.* Harvard University Press, 2000; Getachew, Adom. *Worldmaking After Empire: The Rise and Fall of Self-Determination.* Princeton University Press, 2019.

3. Gilmore, Ruth Wilson. "Forgotten Places and the Seeds of Grassroots Planning." In *Engaging Contradictions: Theory, Politics, and Methods of Activist Scholarship*, edited by Charles R. Hale. University of California Press, 2008, pp. 31–61.

4. Spade, Dean. *Normal Life: Administrative Violence, Critical Trans Politics, and the Limits of Law.* Duke University Press, 2015.

5. Moten, Fred, and Stefano Harney. "The University and the Undercommons: Seven Theses." *Social Text* 22, no. 2 (2004): 101–15.

6. Bendixen, Michala Clante. "How Many Refugees Are Coming to Denmark." *refugees.dk*, July 9, 2024. https://refugees.dk/en/facts/numbers-and-statistics/how-many-are-coming-and-from-where/ [accessed September 2024].

7. Cooper, Melinda. *Family Values: Between Neoliberalism and the New Social Conservatism.* Zone Books, 2019.

8. For more on street-level bureaucrats, see Fox Piven, Frances. "Militant Civil Servants in New York City: Rising Demands of Public Employees Clash with Interest of Blacks in

Our Impoverished Cities." *Trans-Action* 7, no. 1 (November 1969): 24–28; Lipsky, Michael. *Street-Level Bureaucracy: Dilemmas of the Individual in Public Services*. Russell Sage Foundation, 1980.

9. Klein, Naomi. *Doppelganger: A Trip into the Mirror World*. Knopf Canada, 2023.

10. Vartika, Neeraj. "Patents, Pandemics, and the Private Sector: The Battle Over Public Health Norms During COVID-19." *Journal of Public and International Affairs*, May 20, 2022.

11. Fortunati, Leopoldina. *The Arcane of Reproduction*. Autonomedia, 1995; Orozco, Amaia Pérez. *The Feminist Subversion of the Economy: Contributions for Life Against Capital*. Common Notions, 2022.

12. International Labour Organization. *Care Work and Care Jobs for the Future of Decent Work*, 2018.

13. Oxfam International. *Time to Care Report: Unpaid and Underpaid Care Work and the Global Inequality Crisis*, 2020.

14. Mies, Maria. *Patriarchy and Accumulation on a World Scale: Women in the International Division of Labour*. Palgrave Macmillan, 1998; Federici, Silvia. *Caliban and the Witch*. Autonomedia, 2004; Dalla Costa, Mariarosa. *Family, Welfare, and the State: Between Progressivism and the New Deal*. Common Notions, 2015.

15. Gleeson, Jules Joanne, and Elle O'Rourke, eds. *Transgender Marxism*. Pluto Press, 2021, p. 30.

16. Ibid., p. 26.

17. Davies, William. "The New Neoliberalism." *New Left Review*, II, no. 101 (2016): 121–34.

18. Mitropoulos, Angela. *Contract & Contagion: From Biopolitics to Oikonomia*. Minor Compositions, 2013.

19. Fraser, Nancy. "Capitalism's Crisis of Care." *Dissent* 63, no. 4 (2016): 30–37.

20. For more on "surplussed" populations, see Adler-Bolton, Beatrice, and Artie Vierkant. *Health Communism: A Surplus Manifesto*. Verso Books, 2022.

21. Brown, Ashley. "Food Not Bombs Volunteer Found Not Guilty after Citation for Feeding Homeless." *Houston Public Media*, July 31, 2023. https://houstonpublicmedia.org/articles/news/city-of-houston/2023/07/31/458267/food-not-bombs-volunteer-found-not-guilty-after-citation-for-feeding-homeless/ [accessed September 2024]; Dolz, Patricia Ortega. "Spanish Firefighters on Trial for Rescuing Refugees at Sea." *El País English*, May 7, 2018. https://english.elpais.com/elpais/2018/05/07/inenglish/1525676312_002491.html [accessed September 2024]; Lanzillo, Luca. "La Biblioteca comunale di Todi funziona bene? Trasferiamo la direttrice." *AIB WEB*, June 11, 2018. https://aib.it/notizie/trasferimento-bibliotecaria-todi/ [accessed September 2024].

22. Bookchin, Murray. "Libertarian Municipalism: An Overview." *Green Perspectives* 24 (1991): 1–6; Dardot, Pierre, and Christian Laval. *Common: On Revolution in the 21st Century*. Bloomsbury, 2019; Malabou, Catherine. *Il n'y a pas eu de Révolution: Réflexions anarchistes sur la propriété et la condition servile en France*. Rivages, 2024.

23. Graeber, David. *Pirate Enlightenment, or the Real Libertalia*. Farrar, Straus and Giroux, 2023.

24. For the notion of homeplace, see bell hooks. *Yearning: Race, Gender, and Cultural Politics*. South End Press, 1990.

25. For discussions of coercive aspects of care, see Nakano Glenn, Evelyn. *Forced to Care: Coercion*

and Caregiving in America. Harvard University Press, 2010; Lewis, Sophie. *Abolish the Family: A Manifesto for Care and Liberation.* Verso Books, 2022.

26. Mol, Annemarie, Ingunn Moser, and Jeannette Pols, eds. *Care in Practice: On Tinkering in Clinics, Homes and Farms.* transcript Verlag, 2010.

27. Law, John. "Care and Killing: Tensions in Veterinary Practice." In *Care in Practice: On Tinkering in Clinics, Homes and Farms,* p. 69.

28. "David Graeber on Capitalism's Best Kept Secret." *Philonomist,* February 7, 2019. https://philonomist.com/en/entretien/david-graeber-capitalisms-best-kept-secret [accessed September 2024].

29. For ethics of refusal in research, see Ortner, Sherry B. "Resistance and the Problem of Ethnographic Refusal." *Comparative Studies in Society and History* 37, no. 1 (1995): 173–93; Simpson, Audra. "On Ethnographic Refusal: Indigeneity, 'Voice' and Colonial Citizenship." *Junctures,* no. 9 (2007).

30. Bojadžijev, Manuela, and Serhat Karakayalı. "Recuperating the Sideshows of Capitalism: The Autonomy of Migration Today." *e-Flux Journal,* no. 17 (June 2010).

31. La Coalición de Derechos Humanos and No More Deaths. "Disappeared—How the US Border Enforcement Agencies Are Fuelling a Missing Persons Crisis," 2017. http://thedisappearedreport.org/ [accessed September 2024].

32. No More Deaths. "About No More Deaths," February 5, 2021. https://nomoredeaths.org/about-no-more-deaths/ [accessed September 2024].

33. "Ciminalization of Solidarity," *Pirate Care Syllabus*, 2020. https://syllabus.pirate.care/topic/criminalizationofsolidarity/ [accessed September 2024].

34. Firth, Rhiannon. *Disaster Anarchy: Mutual Aid and Radical Action*. Pluto Press, 2022.

35. Linebaugh, Peter, and Marcus Rediker. *The Many-Headed Hydra: Sailors, Slaves, Commoners, and the Hidden History of the Revolutionary Atlantic.* Verso Books, 2000, pp. 160–61.

36. Rediker, Marcus. *Villains of All Nations: Atlantic Pirates in the Golden Age.* Verso Books, 2004, p. 153.

37. Konstam, Angus. *The History of Pirates.* Lyons Press, 1999.

38. Kuhn, Gabriel. *Life Under the Jolly Roger: Reflections on Golden Age Piracy.* PM Press, 2010.

39. Amedeo Policante. *The Pirate Myth.* Routledge, 2015.

40. Sea-Watch. "Sea Rescue as Care." *Pirate Care Syllabus*, 2020. https://syllabus.pirate.care/topic/searescue/ [accessed September 2024].

41. OHCHR. "Statement on Visit to the United Kingdom, by Professor Philip Alston, United Nations Special Rapporteur on Extreme Poverty and Human Rights," November 16, 2018. https://ohchr.org/en/statements/2018/11/statement-visit-united-kingdom-professor-philip-alston-united-nations-special [accessed September 2024].

42. Lewis, Fabian B. "Costly 'Throw-Ups': Electricity Theft and Power Disruptions." *The Electricity Journal* 28, no. 7 (August 1, 2015): 118–35.

43. Zarya, Valentina. "Why Japan's Elderly Are Committing Crimes to 'Break Into Prison.'" *Fortune*, March 28, 2016. https://fortune.

com/2016/03/28/japan-elderly-crime/ [accessed September 2024].

44. Foucault, Michel. *Discipline and Punish*. Random House, 1979.

45. Walia, Harsha. *Undoing Border Imperialism*. AK Press, 2014.

46. Chakelian, Anoosh. "New: You're 23 Times More Likely to Be Prosecuted for Benefit Fraud than Tax Fraud in the UK." *New Statesman*, February 19, 2021. https://newstatesman.com/politics/welfare/2021/02/new-you-re-23-times-more-likely-be-prosecuted-benefit-fraud-tax-fraud-uk [accessed September 2024].

47. Planka.nu. *The Traffic Power Structure*. PM Press, 2016.

48. Docs Not Cops. "Another Key Johnson Claim on the NHS Demolished." *openDemocracy*, October 22, 2019. https://opendemocracy.net/en/ournhs/ournhsanother-key-johnson-claim-nhs-demolished/ [accessed September 2024].

49. Kaplan, Laura. *The Story of Jane: The Legendary Underground Feminist Abortion Service*. University of Chicago Press, 2019.

50. Murphy, Claudette Michelle. *Seizing the Means of Reproduction: Entanglements of Feminism, Health, and Technoscience*. Duke University Press, 2012.

51. As envisioned by psychiatrist and deinstitution-alization advocate Franco Rotelli in 1986 in his "The Invented Institution."

52. More on hacker ethics: Wark, McKenzie. *A Hacker Manifesto*. Harvard University Press, 2004; Forlano, Laura. "Hacking the Feminist Disabled Body." *Journal of Peer Production*, no. 8 (2016).

53. Four Thieves Vinegar Collective. https://fourthievesvinegar.org/.

54. Olesch, Artur. "In the (Good) Hands of Tech." In *Kingdom of the Ill*, eds. Bart van der Heide, Sara Cluggish, and Pavel Pys. Hatje Cantz Verlag, 2022, p. 54.

55. For some pivotal works in ecofeminism, see Merchant, Carolyn. *The Death of Nature: Women, Ecology, and the Scientific Revolution*. HarperCollins, 1990; Plumwood, Val. *Feminism and the Mastery of Nature*. Routledge, 2002; Shiva, Vandana, and Maria Mies. *Ecofeminism*. Zed Books, 2014.

56. Firestone, Shulamith. *The Dialectic of Sex: The Case for Feminist Revolution*. Farrar, Straus and Giroux, 2003; Haraway, Donna. *Simians, Cyborgs and Women: The Reinvention of Nature*. Free Association, 1991; Cuboniks, Laboria. *The Xenofeminist Manifesto: A Politics for Alienation*. Verso Books, 2018; Lewis, Sophie. *Abolish the Family: A Manifesto for Care and Liberation*.

57. Irani, Lilly. "The Cultural Work of Microwork." *New Media & Society* 17, no. 5 (May 1, 2015): 720–39.

58. On "Transhackfeminism" and its quest to repoliticize feminism through biopractice, see Laura Benitez Valero's contribution to the Pirate Care Syllabus. https://syllabus.pirate.care/topic/transhackfeminism/ [accessed September 2024].

59. Chardronnet, Ewen. "GynePunk, the Cyborg Witches of DIY Gynecology." *Makery*, June 30, 2015. https://makery.info/en/2015/06/30/gynepunk-les-sorcieres-cyborg-de-la-gynecologie-diy/ [accessed September 2024].

60. Ibid.

61. Paula Pin, quoted in Ibid.

62. IGLA World. *Trans Legal Mapping Report 2019: Recognition before the Law*, 2019.

63. "Urine Hormone Extraction Action." *Pirate Care Syllabus*, 2020. https://syllabus.pirate.care/session/urinehormoneextractionaction/ [accessed September 2024].

64. Fairy Wings Mutual Aid. "Producing Transdermal Estrogen: A Do-It-Yourself Guide." *CrimethInc.*, December 15, 2022. https://crimethinc.com/2022/12/15/producing-transdermal-estrogen-a-do-it-yourself-guide/ [accessed September 2024].

65. UnfitBit. http://unfitbits.com/ [accessed September 2024].

66. Klein, Naomi. "Screen New Deal. Under Cover of Mass Death, Andrew Cuomo Calls in the Billionaires to Build a High-Tech Dystopia." *The Intercept*, May 8, 2020. https://theintercept.com/2020/05/08/andrew-cuomo-eric-schmidt-coronavirus-tech-shock-doctrine/ [accessed September 2024].

67. Frank's Hospital Workshop. http://frankshospitalworkshop.com/ [accessed September 2024].

68. Marx, Karl. *Capital: A Critique of Political Economy, Volume I. Vol. 35. Karl Marx, Frederick Engels: Collected Works*. Lawrence & Wishart, 2010.

69. Wark, McKenzie. *Molecular Red: Theory for the Anthropocene*. Verso Books, 2015.

70. Wajcman, Judy. *TechnoFeminism*. Polity, 2004. Cockburn, Cynthia, and Ruža First-Dilić. *Bringing Technology Home: Gender and Technology in a Changing Europe*. Open University Press, 1994. Bailey, Moya. *Misogynoir Transformed*. New York University Press, 2021.

71. Safi, Michael. "Oxford/AstraZeneca Covid Vaccine Research 'Was 97% Publicly Funded'." *Guardian*, April 15, 2021. https://theguardian.com/science/2021/apr/15/oxfordastrazeneca-covid-vaccine-research-was-97-publicly-funded [accessed September 2024].

72. Spade, Dean. *Mutual Aid: Building Solidarity During This Crisis (and the Next)*. Verso Books, 2020. Sitrin, M., and Colectiva Sembrar, eds. *Pandemic Solidarity. Mutual Aid During the COVID-19 Crisis*. Pluto Press, 2020; Bringel, Breno, and Geoffrey Pleyers, eds. *Social Movements and Politics during COVID-19*. Bristol University Press, 2022.

73. Colau, Ada, and Adrià Alemany. *Mortgaged Lives*. Journal of Aesthetics and Protest Press/Herbst, 2014.

74. Ginty, Timothy. "The PAH: Defending the Right to Housing in Spain." *ROAR Magazine*, July 23, 2015. https://roarmag.org/essays/pah-human-right-housing-spain/ [accessed September 2024].

75. Adell, Miquel, Anna Lara, and Elvi Mármol. "La PAH: Origen, Evolución y Rumbo." *Anuario de Movimientos Sociales* (2013): 1–20.

76. Adkins, Lisa, Melinda Cooper, and Martijn Konings. *The Asset Economy*. Wiley, 2020, p. 69ff.

77. Sebály, Bernadett. "'We All Have to Live Somewhere!' The Hungarian Housing Movement—a Bottom-up View—1989–2021." *Lefteast*, June 15, 2022. https://lefteast.org/we-all-have-to-live-somewhere-the-hungarian-housing-movement-a-bottom-up-view-1989-2021/ [accessed September 2024].

78. "Tech and Science in the Time of COVID-19." *Pirate Care Syllabus*. 2020. https://syllabus.

pirate.care/session/techandcorona/ [accessed September 2024].

79. Bruno Ramirez. "Self-reduction of Prices in Italy." In *Midnight Oil: Work, Energy, War, 1973–1992*, edited by Midnight Notes. Autonomedia, 1992, p. 92.

80. Ibid., p. 86.

81. Trogal, Kim. "Confronting Unjust Urban Infrastructures: Repairing Water Connections as Acts of Care." In *Pirate Care Conference*. Centre for Postdigital Cultures, University of Coventry, 2019.

82. Redecker, Eva von. "Ownership's Shadow: Neoauthoritarianism as Defense of Phantom Possession." *Critical Times* 3, no. 1 (April 1, 2020): 33–67; Ferreira da Silva, Denise. "The Racial Limits of Social Justice: The Ruse of Equality of Opportunity and the Global Affirmative Action Mandate." *Critical Ethnic Studies* 2, no. 2 (2016).

83. Pomeranz, Kenneth. *The Great Divergence: China, Europe, and the Making of the Modern World Economy*. Princeton University Press, 2000.

84. Haraway, Donna. "Anthropocene, Capitalocene, Plantationocene, Chthulucene: Making Kin." *Environmental Humanities* 6, no. 1 (May 1, 2015): 159–65.

85. Park, K.-Sue. "Race and Property Law," 2021. https://papers.ssrn.com/sol3/papers.cfm?abstract_id=3908102/ [accessed September 2024]; Nichols, Robert. *Theft Is Property!: Dispossession and Critical Theory*. Duke University Press, 2019; Malabou, Catherine. *Il n'y a pas eu de Révolution*.

86. Shiva, Vandana. *The Enclosure and Recovery of the Commons: Biodiversity, Indigenous Knowledge, and*

Intellectual Property Rights. Research Foundation for Science, Technology, and Ecology, 1997.

87. "Open Source Seed Initiative—About," December 8, 2014. https://osseeds.org/about/ [accessed September 2024].

88. Cangiano, Serena, and Zoe Romano. "Ease of Repair as a Design Ideal: A Reflection on How Open Source Models Can Support Longer Lasting Ownership of, and Care for, Technology." *ephemera* 19, no. 2 (2019): 441–9.

89. Koebler, Jason. "Why American Farmers Are Hacking Their Tractors With Ukrainian Firmware." *Vice*, March 21, 2017. https://vice.com/en/article/xykkkd/why-american-farmers-are-hacking-their-tractors-with-ukrainian-firmware [accessed September 2024].

90. "#StandingRockSyllabus." *NYC Stands with Standing Rock*, October 11, 2016. https://nycstandswithstandingrock.wordpress.com/standingrocksyllabus/ [accessed September 2024].

91. Stengers, Isabelle. *In Catastrophic Times: Resisting the Coming Barbarism.* Open Humanities Press, 2015, p. 85.

92. Johnson, Richard. "Really Useful Knowledge." In *CCCS Selected Working Papers: Volume 1*, no. 1. Routledge, 2014, pp. 751–77.

93. Swartz, Aaron. "Guerilla Open Access Manifesto." July 2008. https://archive.org/stream/GuerillaOpenAccessManifesto/Goamjuly2008_djvu.txt/ [accessed September 2024].

94. Custodians.online. "In Solidarity with Library Genesis and Sci-hub," November 30, 2015. http://custodians.online/ [accessed September 2024].

95. Suresh, Akhilesh. "University of Oxford vs. Rameshwari Photocopy Services." *Supremo Amicus* 23 (2021): 585.

96. American Library Association. "An Open Letter to America's Publishers from ALA President Maureen Sullivan." *Text. News and Press Center*, September 28, 2012. https://ala.org/news/2012/09/open-letter-america's-publishers-ala-president-maureen-sullivan [accessed September 2024].

97. Curcic, Dimitrije. "Academic Publishers Statistics—WordsRated," June 21, 2023. https://wordsrated.com/academic-publishers-statistics/ [accessed September 2024].

98. Larivière, Vincent, Stefanie Haustein, and Philippe Mongeon. "The Oligopoly of Academic Publishers in the Digital Era." *PLoS ONE* 10, no. 6 (June 10, 2015).

99. Liang, Lawrence. "Shadow Libraries." *e-flux Journal*, no. 37 (September 2012). http://e-flux.com/journal/37/61228/shadow-libraries/ [accessed September 2024].

100. Himmelstein, Daniel, Ariel Rodriguez Romero, Jacob Levernier, Thomas Anthony Munro, Stephen Reid McLaughlin, Bastian Greshake Tzovaras, and Casey S. Greene. "Sci-Hub Provides Access to Nearly All Scholarly Literature." *eLife* 7 (2018).

101. Elbakyan, Alexandra. "Why Science Is Better with Communism? The Case of Sci-Hub." In *UNT Open Access Symposium*, Denton, TX. May 19–20, 2016. https://digital.library.unt.edu/ark:/67531/metadc850001/ [accessed September 2024].

102. Custodians.online [accessed September 2024].

103. Ferrer, Francisco. *The Origin and Ideals of the Modern School*. Watts, 2013, pp. 32–3.

104. Malaguzzi, Loris. *Fragments I. Commentaries for a Code to Reading the Exhibition.* Reggio Emilia, Reggio Children, 2020, p. 18.

105. Harney, Stefano, and Fred Moten. *The Undercommons: Fugitive Planning & Black Study.* Autonomedia, 2013, p. 26.

106. Academic Freedom Index 2022. https://academic-freedom-index.net/ [accessed September 2024].

107. Capuzzi, Lucia. "Afghanistan. Sotto i taleban lezioni alle donne della scuola «che non c'è»." *Avvenire*, June 29, 2023. https://avvenire.it/mondo/pagine/sotto-i-taleban-lezioni-di-giornalismo-alle-donne-della-scuola-che-non-c/ [accessed September 2024].

108. Fragnito, Maddalena, ed. Como Aprire Un Nido Pirata Nel Quartiere, 2019. https://soprasottomilano.it/come-aprire-un-nido-pirata-nel-quartiere/ [accessed September 2024].

109. Zechner, Manuela. *Commoning Care & Collective Power: Childcare Commons and the Micropolitics of Municipalism in Barcelona.* transversal texts, 2019.

110. Dokuzović, Lina and The Yard Movement. "Navigating Dangerous Terrain: The Yard Movement and the Tactics of Publishing, Care, and Collectivity of the Belarusian Museum of Stones." *transversal* podcast, 2023. https://transversal.at/audio/navigating-dangerous-terrain [accessed September 2024].

111. Ibid.

112. Chiaramonte, Xenia. *Governare il conflitto: La criminalizzazione del movimento No Tav.* Mimesis, 2019.

113. Epstein, Steven. "The Construction of Lay Expertise: AIDS Activism and the Forging of

Credibility in the Reform of Clinical Trials." *Science, Technology, & Human Values* 20, no. 4 (October 1995): 408–37.

114. Graeber. *Pirate Enlightenment, or the Real Libertalia.*

115. Orozco. *The Feminist Subversion of the Economy.*

116. Beard, Lisa. *If We Were Kin: Race, Identification, and Intimate Political Appeals.* Oxford University Press, 2023.

117. James, Sandy, Jody Herman, Susan Rankin, Mara Keisling, Lisa Mottet, and Ma'ayan Anafi. "The Report of the 2015 US Transgender Survey." *National Center for Transgender Equality*, 2016.

118. Shepard, Benjamin. "From Community Organization to Direct Services: The Street Trans Action Revolutionaries to Sylvia Rivera Law Project." *Journal of Social Service Research* 39, no. 1 (January 1, 2013): 95–114.

119. Blanchard, Sessi Kuwabara. "At STAR House, Marsha P. Johnson and Sylvia Rivera Created a Home for Trans People." *Vice*, June 8, 2020. https://vice.com/en/article/z3enva/star-house-sylvia-rivera-marsha-p-johnson [accessed September 2024].

120. hooks. *Yearning: Race, Gender, and Cultural Politics.*

121. Hill Collins, Patricia. *Black Feminist Thought.* Routledge, 2000; Naples, Nancy A. "Activist Mothering: Cross-Generational Continuity in the Community Work of Women from Low-Income Urban Neighborhoods." *Gender & Society* 6, no. 3 (September 1992): 441–63.

122. Talaga, Tanya. *Seven Fallen Feathers: Racism, Death, and Hard Truths in a Northern City.* House of Anansi Press Incorporated, 2017.

123. Browne, Simone. *Dark Matters: On the Surveillance of Blackness.* Duke University Press, 2015.

124. O'Brien, M. E. *Family Abolition: Capitalism and the Communizing of Care.* Pluto Press, 2023.

125. Wacquant, Loic. "Resolving the Trouble with 'Race.'" *New Left Review*, no. 133/134 (April 13, 2022): 67–88.

126. Thornton also wrote up her vision in another VAGABONDS book, *The Hologram: Feminist, Peer-to-Peer Health for a Post-Pandemic Future.* Pluto Press, 2020, but also contributed a topic on *The Hologram: A Peer-to-Peer Social Technology of Care* to our Pirate Care Syllabus. https://syllabus.pirate.care/topic/hologramsocialcare/ [accessed September 2024].

127. Power Makes us Sick (PMS). https://powermakesussick.noblogs.org/ [accessed September 2024].

128. Economic Commission for Latin America and the Caribbean. *Femicidal Violence in Figures Bulletin,* 2022. https://cepal.org/en/publications/type/femicidal-violence-figures-latin-america-and-caribbean [accessed September 2024].

129. Acción Directa Autogestiva, quoted in: Cornelia Sollfrank, ed. *The Beautiful Warriors. Technofeminist Praxis in the Twenty-first Century.* Minor Compositions, 2019, p. 39.

130. The Autodefensas Hackfeministas. https://lab-interconectividades.net/autodefensas-hackfeministas/ [accessed September 2024].

131. See the work of Gesturing Decolonial Futures Collective. https://decolonialfutures.net/.

132. Pressenza. "Pia Klemp Refuses the Grand Vermeil Medal Awarded to Her by the City of Paris," August 21, 2019. https://pressenza.com/2019/08/pia-klemp-refuses-the-grand-vermeil-medal-awarded-to-her-by-the-city-of-paris/ [accessed September 2024].

133. Linebaugh and Rediker. *The Many-Headed Hydra.*

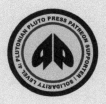

Thanks to our Patreon subscriber:

Ciaran Kane

Who has shown generosity and comradeship in support of our publishing.

The Pluto Press Newsletter

Hello friend of Pluto!

Want to stay on top of the best radical books we publish?

Then sign up to be the first to hear about our new books, as well as special events, podcasts and videos.

You'll also get 50% off your first order with us when you sign up.

Come and join us!

Go to bit.ly/PlutoNewsletter